Return circulation and Norepinephrine : an update

In order to respect the publication schedule, I did the modifications requested by the editor and the proof corrections.
I hope authors will not mind too much and will excuse me if odd mistakes appear in their texts. Thank you very much.

J. Daver M.D.Ph. D.
Science et Communication

Return circulation and Norepinephrine : an update

Proceedings of the 3rd International Symposium held in Cairo (Egypt) March 12-17th, 1990

Editor
P.M. Vanhoutte

Pierre Fabre

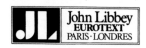

British Library Cataloguing in Publication Data
Return circulation and norepinephrine : an update.
1. Humans. Veins. Diseases
I. Vanhoutte, P.M. (Paul M)
616.14

ISBN 0 86196 293-1

Editions John Libbey Eurotext
6 rue Blanche, 92120 Montrouge, France.
Tél. : (1) 47 35 85 52
Fax : (1) 46.57.10.09

John Libbey and Company Ltd
13 Smiths Yard, Summerley Street, London SW18 4HR, England.
Tél. : (81) 947.27.77

John Libbey CIC
Via L. Spallanzani, 11, 00161 Rome, Italy
Tél. : (06) 862.289

Contents

Preface

This volume contains the proceedings of a symposium held in Cairo and devoted to the pharmacology and pathophysiology of the post-capillary circulation. It is the third in a series devoted to the same theme. The first two meetings were held in Athens in 1983 and in Sorrento in 1987. As in Athens, the meeting held in Sorrento provided an opportunity for scientists and clinicians to compare their views on the venous circulation.

In Athens the clinical topics comprised essentially a number of relatively basic data aimed at demonstrating the interest of venotonic therapy. A main concern at the time was for the pharmaceutical industry to justify the commercialization of specific products intended to treat the disorders provoked by chronic venous insufficiency. The meeting provided a setting in which to demonstrate, at the clinical level, the validity of a number of fundamental concepts emerging from basic pharmacological studies. The essential contribution of this meeting has been to revalorize the veins (no less noble than the arteries to borrow the words of a journalist summing up the meeting).

In Sorrento the clinical studies presented constituted a second generation of investigations attempting to meet the standards of regulatory approval within the context of the EEC norms. The studies presented in Sorrento embraced three major themes.

The first theme was venous insufficiency of the lower limbs. The two double blind placebo controlled studies that were presented are now complemented by comparative studies. The second theme dealt with contraceptive metrorrhagia, be it caused by intrauterine devices or by oral contraceptives. These gynaecological themes will be also expanded in these proceedings to the premenstrual syndrome. The third theme covered discussed venous dysfunction in haemorrhoids. A major achievement in Sorrento was the demonstration by plethysmography in people, that the venous consequences of local heating in peripheral veins are identical to the effects described *in vitro* in animal cutaneous veins. Hence the clinical studies reported in Sorrento explained the renewed outbreak of vein disorders in summer and why excessive heating in winter may give rise to venous dysfunction.

This volume, as the reader will see, is the logical continuation of the two previous ones. It sums up the impact of the various factors on the return circulation to the heart that have received particular attention in the last three years. First, studies will be presented on the impact of estrogens on the veins. From a pharmacological point of view the facilitatory role of estrogens on adrenergic responses is fairly well established.

Clinical studies included in this volume will attempt to achieve a clear overview in the clinical context of the interactions between the different hormonal systems and venous function. Another major accent of the Cairo meeting was to focus on the lymphatic system, not only as a contributor to venous disease, but also as a key player in the side effects of commonly prescribed cardiovascular drugs.

Thus, from the clinical point of view, the inhibition of the lymphatic pump by Ca^{++}-antagonists provides a partial explanation for the edema frequently observed with these agents. The discussion in Cairo provided encouraging data for the management of this side effect. A third major theme, developed in this volume, are the increased efforts to correlate histological and biochemical alterations of the pathological venous wall, whether in aging or after denervation.

A last, overall important topic covered is the microcirculation and how its disorders may explain certain symptoms associated with venous disease. With these different themes, this volume represents a true update of the current knowledge of the postcapillary circulation and its abnormalities that lead to, or accompany chronic venous insufficiency. It provides a renewed platform for the understanding of the beneficial therapeutic effect of venotonic agents. As such, it should become an important tool not only for pharmacologists and pathologists, but also for the practitioner who tries to treat venous disease medically.

P.M. Vanhoutte

Return circulation and Norepinephrine : an update. Ed. P.M. Vanhoutte. John Libbey Eurotext, Paris © 1991, pp. 1-14.

1

Venous wall and venous disease

P.M. Vanhoutte

Center for Experimental Therapeutics, Baylor College of Medicine, Houston, Texas, USA

Introduction

This chapter summarizes current thinking on the role of the limb veins in thermoregulatory and gravitational adjustments. It updates earlier overviews of the function of the venous wall in health and disease [1-5]. The reader is referred to these previous overviews for details and earlier references.

Physiology

The major components of the vein wall are collagen, elastin, and smooth muscle. Leg veins contain more smooth muscle than do arm veins, and in both the arm and the leg superficial veins contain more muscle than deep veins. These differences are in keeping with the higher hydrostatic pressure in the lower extremities and the more active role played by the cutaneous veins. The venous wall is very distensible. This means that minimal increases in distending pressure can potentially cause venous pooling. The distensibility of the normal venous wall is limited by its collagen structure and by the contraction of its venous smooth muscle [1-5].

The effective venous distending pressure (transmural pressure) is determined by the pressure of the blood within the vein minus the counterpressure exerted by the surrounding tissues. The venous blood pressure depends on : (a) the arterial pressure and the diameter of the arterioles. When the arterioles dilate, the venous pressure is augmented ; (b) the hydrostatic load, which is dependent on gravitational forces ; and (c) the pressure in the downstream part of the low-pressure system [1-5].

The most common gravitational stress for the human occurs when he/she changes from the supine to the standing position. When lying, the hydrostatic load is nearly the same for all parts of the body, and the pressures within the blood vessels depend on the force generated by the heart. Large hydrostatic gradients occur on standing *(Figure 1)*. In the abdomen the increase in venous hydrostatic pressure is balanced by the increased tissue pressure exerted by the abdominal viscera. This places the splanchnic veins in an ideal position for modulation of vascular capacity. In the dependent extremities the arterial and venous pressures are increased to the same extent by the hydrostatic load, so there are no changes in the driving force to flow *(Figure 2)* [1-5].

The increased pressure in the limb veins, however, has two consequences. One is to increase capillary pressure, causing increased filtration. The other

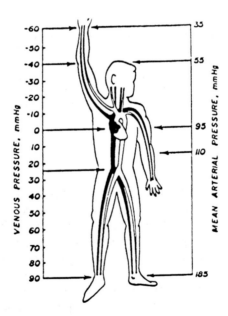

Figure 1. – Arterial and venous pressures in the motionless, standing subject. Influence of hydrostatic pressure on the columns of blood in the arteries (open vessels) and veins (solid vessels). (From reference 2, by permission).

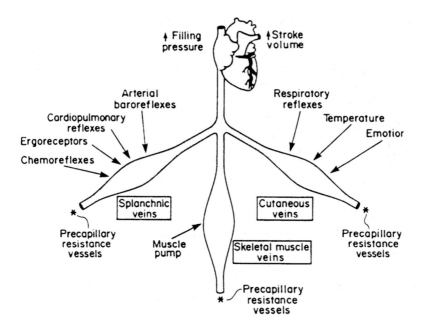

Figure 2. – Regulation of the systemic venous system. The three main components of this system are the splanchnic, the skeletal muscles and the cutaneous veins. The splanchnic capacitance (spleen, liver, gastrointestine) is controlled predominantly by the cardiovascular reflexes; the veins in the skeletal muscles by the skeletal muscle pump and the cutaneous veins by the thermoregulatory centers, by emotion and by respiratory reflexes. These regulatory mechanisms act to control the amount of blood in the systemic veins relative to that in the heart and lungs. Thus they have a vital role in adjusting the filling pressure of the heart and the stroke volume. The cutaneous veins have a key role in body temperature regulation. (From reference 5, by permission).

is to cause pooling of blood at the venous side. The accumulation of blood in the limb veins is limited by the collagen fibers of the venous wall and by the presence of venous valves, which subdivide the venous blood column into segments *(Figure 3)*. The pressure inside these segments is less than would occur if the valves were absent. If the standing is prolonged, the maintained hydrostatic load above the proximal venous valves causes the insufficiency, and this process continues until the most distal valves become insufficient. At this time, the venous pressure in the foot approximates the pressure of a column of blood extending vertically from the foot to the heart and hence may approach 90 mm Hg. As a consequence, several hundred milliliters of blood accumulate in the lower extremities [1-5].

3

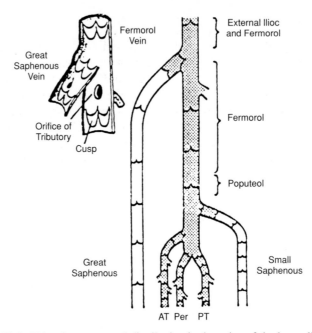

Figure 3. – *Right:*Valve frequency and distribution in the veins of the lower limb. Stippled = deep veins. Clear = superficial veins. AT = Anterior tibial. Per = peroneal. PT = posterior tibial. *Left:*Upper portions of the fermoral and great (long) saphenous veins laid open to show valves. (From reference 2, by permission).

In people, venous valves are more prominent in the veins of the leg than the arm, reflecting the adaptation to larger changes in hydrostatic pressure. Each valve possesses two cusps composed of endothelium-covered collagen. They are found in the superficial and deep venous systems of the leg, as well as in the branches connecting these two systems. In the latter they are designed to permit blood to flow from the superficial to the deep veins *(Figure 3)*. This arrangement of valves allows the massaging action of contracting skeletal muscle to propel blood toward the heart in the upright posture (muscle pump). Indeed, the peripheral pooling of blood on standing may be counteracted effectively by the massaging action of the leg muscles during their contractions. During the latter the veins within the muscles are compressed, the pressure distending them decreases; the competency of the valves is restored, and the long hydrostatic column again is broken into shorter segments. The decrease in pressure in deep veins allows blood to flow into them from the superficial veins through communicating branches; hence, the pressure in the cutaneous veins also decreases [1-5].

Venous smooth muscle

The distensibility of the venous wall is affected considerably by the degree of contraction of the smooth muscle that it contains *(Figure 4)*. Venous smooth muscle cells have the basic structure and functional characteristics of vascular smooth muscle cells. They contain the usual organelles of contractile tissue including contractile proteins (actin and myosin), surface vesicles, sarcoplasmic reticulum and mitochondria [1-4, 7]. The amount of smooth muscle varies with the splanchnic veins and the cutaneous veins being the most richly endowed, which is in line with their role as active capacitance

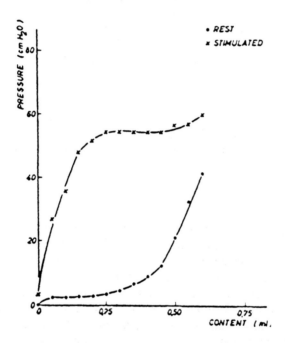

Figure 4. – The venous wall is very distensible, as demonstrated in an isolated segment of canine cutaneous vein. The intraluminal pressure (ordinate) is recorded and the content is increased by infusing a known amount (abscissa) of physiological salt solution. Important changes in volume are accommodated for minimal changes in intraluminal pressure, until the stiffer components (collagen) of the venous wall are stretched (●———●). The responses of the venous smooth muscle also depend on the degree of distension. This is illustrated by the changing increases in pressure generated at different distension levels, by electrical stimulation (15 Hz for 10s; x———x) of the adrenergic nerve endings in the venous wall. Thus, activation of the adrenergic nerves considerably reduces the distensibility of the venous wall. (From reference 6, by permission).

5

and thermoregulatory blood vessels, respectively. The contraction of venous smooth muscle is triggered by increases in the cytoplasmic Ca^{2+} concentration which set the actomyosin interaction in motion. The Ca^{2+} can originate from the extracellular space and enters the cells (calcium entry), presumably though specific calcium channels. These channels are either opened by changes in cell membrane potential (potential-operated calcium channels) or by the interaction of a vasoconstrictor agonist with its receptors on the cell membrane (receptor-operated calcium channels). The activator Ca^{2+} can also be mobilized from cellular stores (internal side of the cell membrane, sarcoplasmic reticulum) *(Figure 5)*. The relative importance of these sources of Ca^{2+} ions varies among venous smooth muscle of different anatomical origin. Thus, splanchnic venous smooth muscle relies mainly on the entry of Ca^{2+} to trigger the contractile process, while in cutaneous venous smooth muscle cellular mobilization of the activator ion plays a major role in excitation-contraction coupling. At the end of the activation period, the Ca^{2+} is removed from the cytoplasm wither to the cellular stores or to the extracellular fluid [1-4, 8].

In most veins, contractions of the smooth muscle are caused by the presence in the vicinity of the cells of neurohumoral mediators. Among those, the catecholamines, particularly norepinephrine liberated from adrenergic nerve endings, play the major role. Catecholamines cause contraction of venous smooth muscle by activation of α-adrenergic receptors of the smooth muscle cells (post-junctional α-adrenoceptors) that belong to two subtypes : α_1-adrenoceptors, which resemble those found in most arterial smooth muscle, and α_2-adrenergic receptors, with pharmacological properties comparable to those of the prejunctional (presynaptic) α-adrenoceptors found on adrenergic nerve endings [5, 8-15]. In cutaneous veins, the norepinephrine released from adrenergic nerves appears to activate preferentially the postjunctional adrenoceptors of the α_2-subtype (5, 16, 17). In these veins α-adrenergic activation causes contraction mainly by mobilizing cellular Ca^{2+} [5]. The adrenergic nerve endings in veins are endowed with both inhibitory and prejunctional receptors [18-23], the functional role of these receptors is unknown [1-5].

The evidence available indicates that most peripheral veins, if innervated, receive only adrenergic neurons. Hormonal regulators such as angiotensin II and vasopressin have little direct effect on venous smooth muscle cells. By contrast, in most vascular beds, locally produced autacoids (histamine, 5-hydroxytryptamine, kinins, certain prostaglandins and endothelins) cause constriction of venules and veins, which promotes the exudation of fluid and contributes to the local edema that these compounds produce [1-5, 24, 25].

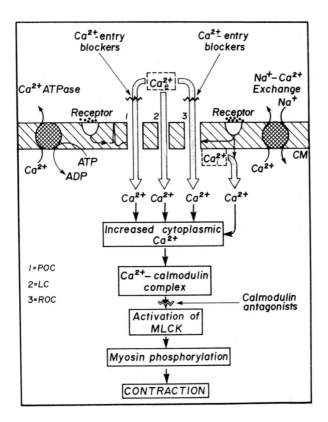

Figure 5. – Calcium-dependent regulation of contractile activity in vascular smooth muscle. Cytoplasmic calcium (Ca^{2+}) levels are increased by calcium influx through potential-operated calcium channels (1, POC), a passive calcium 'leak' channel (2, LC, calcium entry that occurs under resting conditions) and receptor-operated calcium channels (3, ROC). Receptor-occupation by a specific agonist may also induce release of calcium from intracellular storage sites or may depolarize the cell membrane and activate the potential-operated channel. Calcium activates myosin light chain kinase (MLCK) by binding to calmodulin. Activated myosin light chain kinase catalyses the phosphorylation of myosin, which increases actin-myosin interactions, resulting in contraction. Cytoplasmic calcium levels are reduced through the operation of cell membrane (CM) pumps, including Ca^{2+}-ATPase (left) and a Na^{+}-Ca^{2+} countertransport (right) that promote calcium efflux (From reference 5, by permission).

Sympathetic nervous control

The degree of adrenergic innervation of the veins varies widely. Cutaneous and splanchnic veins are most densely innervated; the large conduit veins and the deep limb veins, in particular those draining skeletal muscles, receive only a sparse adrenergic innervation. Thus, active neurogenically-mediated changes in venous diameter occur mainly in the skin and the splanchnic area; other veins play mainly a passive role although they can constrict in unison with the cutaneous and splanchnic veins when the levels of circulating catecholamines augment [1-5, 26-28].

The sympathetic control of the cutaneous veins is dominated by the hypothalamic thermoregulatory centers, which, when the body temperature decreases, augment the sympathetic outflow to the skin; a rise in body temperature induces opposite changes [1-5].

Local control

When venous smooth muscle is activated, its actual constrictor response will be determined in part by the local conditions to which it is exposed. Thus, changes in distending pressure not only cause passive mobilization or pooling of blood, but, as a consequence of the altered distension level, also shift the smooth muscle cells of the venous wall along their length-active tension relationship, and thus augment the resistance to distension of the venous wall *(Figure 4)* [1-5].

Variations in local temperature profoundly affect the responsiveness of venous smooth muscle, albeit in opposite direction in cutaneous and deep veins. As said before, the smooth muscle of cutaneous veins contains post-junctional α_1- and α_2-adrenoceptors. The norepinephrine released from adrenergic nerve endings activates preferentially the post-junctional α_2-adrenoceptors; exogenous norepinephrine activates both subtypes. Local warming reduces, and local cooling augments markedly, the cutaneous venoconstriction caused by stimulation of the sympathetic nerves; these effects of local changes in temperature are less pronounced during constrictions evoked by exogenous norepinephrine. The modulation in adrenergic responsiveness caused by cooling and warming are due primarily to an increase and decrease, respectively, of the reactivity of the post-junctional α_2-adrenoceptors. Local cooling inhibits the responsiveness to α_1-adrenergic activation. However, if the α_1-adrenergic stimulus is evoked by a full agonist (e.g. norepinephrine, phenylephrine), the large α_1-adrenoceptor reserve, characteristic of the cutaneous veins, buffers the inhibitory effect of cold. This allows the expression of the augmented responsiveness to α_2-adrenergic activation, in particular during sympathetic nerve stimulation *(Figure 6)* [1-5, 29, 30]. The modulation, by changes in temperature, of the response to sympathetic activation may involve transmitters other than norepinephrine, in particular ATP released together with norepinephrine. In contrast to the cutaneous veins, cooling depresses the responsiveness of the smooth muscle cells of the deep veins [1-5, 29, 30]. The adrenergic nerves release not only norepinephrine,

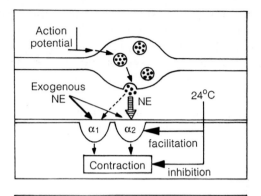

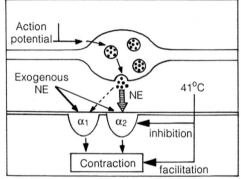

Figure 6. – Effects of temperature on adrenergic neuroeffector interaction in canine cutaneous veins. α, postjunctional α-adrenoceptor; NE, norepinephrine. (From reference 5, by permission).

but also adenosine triphosphate (ATP), which causes contraction of venous smooth muscle; the response is augmented by cooling [31, 32].

The cutaneous venoconstriction caused by local cooling limits the physical heat loss, and directs the superficial blood toward the deep veins, which dilate because the blood returning from the skin is cold. This dilatation results in a decreased flow velocity and promotes counter-current heat exchange with the arterial blood running alongside the deep veins. Thus, the cold blood is partly rewarmed before re-entering the body core [1-5].

Endothelium

Although in arteries the endothelium mediates relaxation to a variety of endogenous neurohumoral vasodilators, endothelium-dependent relaxations are less pronounced in veins because their endothelial cells are poor releasers of endothelium-derived relaxing factor (EDRF). Actually, in veins, the endothelium tends to generate vasoconstrictor substances (endothelium-derived contracting factor; EDCF). Venous smooth muscle is exquisitely sensitive to the constrictor effect of the endothelium-derived peptide, endothelin. The reasons for the heterogeneity in endothelium-dependent responses between arteries and veins are unknown; they may include chronic exposure to different flows and/or blood with a relatively low oxygen content [25, 33-36].

Varicose veins

Varicose veins are due to abnormal distensibility of the connective tissue in the vein wall. All limb veins from patients with varicosities are more distensible than normal, indicating the genetic basis for the abnormality. The fact that they occur in the legs illustrates that increased hydrostatic pressure is a major external factor precipitating their occurrence [1-5].

The varicosities usually start in the superficial veins at the points where the communicating veins originate. The increased distensibility of the wall renders the valves incompetent, which causes the backflow of blood. The combination of the retrograde flow in the superficial veins and in the communicating branches causes the typical tortuous pattern of the varicosities. The increased transmural pressure in the postcapillary vessels favors the exudation of fluid and edema formation. The poor tissue drainage causes ischemia, which favors inflammation, infection, thrombosis, and tissue damage (ulcer). The valvular incompetence associated with varicose veins renders the muscle pump less effective *(Figure 7),* [1-5].

The cause of primary varicose veins is uncertain. Genetic factors probably are a major determinant, and a person who has close relatives with varicose veins runs an increased risk of developing this disease. Isolated strips from human varicose veins are more distensible than are similar preparations from normal subjects ; the sensitivity of the smooth muscle cells to vasoactive agents seems unchanged, and the defect is probably due to the presence of abnormal or immature connective tissue in the vein wall. The presence of mucopolysaccharides increases the resistance to stretch of both collagen and elastin fibers. The activity of lysosomal enzymes that interfere with the metabolism of mucopolysaccharides is significantly higher in varicose than in normal human saphenous veins ; this could be the origin of the abnormal physical properties of the vein wall [1-5].

In most statistical studies of the occurrence of varicose veins, the anomaly appears to be more frequent in women than in men. During the menstrual cycle, there are cyclic changes ; venous distensibility seems to increase with

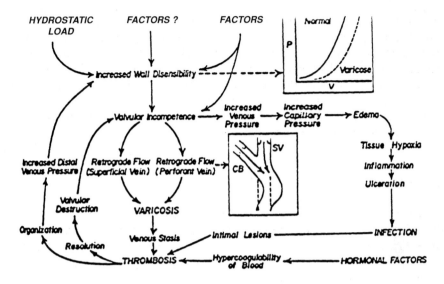

Figure 7. – Sequence of events in the development of varicose veins and venous thrombosis. The distensibility of the wall of veins from patients with varicose veins is greater than normal, and for each increase in hydrostatic pressure (P) the veins accommodate a larger volume of blood (V : upper inset). The increased distention causes the incompetence of the venous valves of the superficial veins (SV) and the communicating branches (CB) with the deep veins (lower inset). The retrograde flows cause the tortuous pattern of the varicose veins. (From reference 2, by permission).

the level of progesterone. During pregnancy the distensibility of the forearm veins is augmented, and the increase is more pronounced in women suffering from varicosities prior to pregnancy. These factors together with the increase in hydrostatic load caused by the gravid uterus compressing the pelvic veins may explain why varices frequently occur first during pregnancy. Increased venous distensibility has also been reported during prolonged administration of oral contraceptives. These drugs have been claimed to facilitate the occurrence of venous thrombosis; if this happens, it may be due to interference with the coagulation mechanism [1-5, 37].

Venotonic therapy

Of the different drugs proposed to increase peripheral venous tone, the author's laboratory has had the most experience with the extract of *Ruscus acu-*

11

leatus. It causes contraction of isolated cutaneous veins, due to activation of both postjunctional alpha$_1$- and alpha$_2$-adrenergic receptors, by releasing endogenous norepinephrine from the adrenergic nerve endings, and through a direct action on the venous smooth muscle *(Figure 8)* [38-41]. The contractions caused by the extract are augmented by local warming and reduced by cooling, because the active principle acts as a partial alpha1-adrenergic agonist whereby the modulating effect of temperature is not buffered by a receptor-reserve [29, 30, 39]. The *in vitro* thermosensitivity of the venoconstrictor effect of *Ruscus* permits to predict that the drug will retain its therapeutic effect in the face of an augmented ambient temperature, a condition which favors the occurrence of venous pooling in the limbs [1-5]). Recent observations in animals treated chronically with progesterone (which is another factor believed to favor the occurrence of venous disease [1-5]), indicate that the hormone potentiates the direct constrictor effect of *Ruscus* on venous smooth muscle (Miller and Vanhoutte, unpublished observations). If this were to occur in people, it also may help to explain the beneficial effect of *Ruscus* in patients with varicose veins.

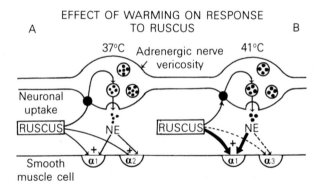

Figure 8. – Proposed mechanisms of action for *Ruscus* (α = α-adrenoceptors). A, normal conditions; B, warming. NE = norepinephrine, α = α-adrenoceptor. (From reference 41, by permission).

References

1. Shepherd JT, Vanhoutte PM. Veins and their control. W. B. Saunders Co., London-Philadelphia, 1975; pp 1-269.

2. Shepherd JT, Vanhoutte PM. The Human Cardiovascular System. Facts and Concepts. Raven Press, New York, 1979; pp. 1-315.

3. Vanhoutte PM. Role of the veins in the circulation. Acta Cardiol 1981; 36 : 239-248.

4. Vanhoutte PM. Control of venous function. Int Angiol 1984;3 (suppl.) : 40-46.

5. Vanhoutte PM. The role of the systemic veins : an update, Phlebology 1988;3, Suppl. 1 : 13-25.

6. Vanhoutte PM, Leusen I. The reactivity of isolated venous preparations to electric stimulation. Pfuegers Arch, 1969; 306 : 341-353.

7. Wang Z, Stephens NL. Normally cycling and latch bridges in venous smooth muscle. Blood Vessels 1989; 26 : 272-279.

8. Sjoberg T, Andersson KE, Norgren L, *et al*. Comparative effects of some calcium-channel blockers on human peripheral arteries and veins. Acta Physiol Scand 1987; 130 : 419-427.

9. Elsner D, Stewart DJ, Sommer 0, *et al*. Postsynaptic α_1- and α_2-adrenergic receptors in adrenergic control of capacitance vessel tone *in vivo*. Hypertension 1986; 8 : 1003-1014

10. Flavahan NA, Vanhoutte PM. Heterogeneity of alpha-adrenergic responsiveness in vascular smooth muscle : Role of receptor subtypes and receptor reserve. *In "The Alpha-l Adrenergic Receptors"*, Ed : Ruffolo, R.R. The Humana Press, Inc. 1987;351-403.

11. Itoh H, Kohli JD, Rajferf SI. Pharmacological characterization of the postsynaptic alpha-adrenoceptors in isolated canine mesenteric arteries and veins. Naunyn-Schmiedeberg's Arch Pharmacol 1987; 335 : 44-49.

12. Sjöberg T, Steen S, Skarby T, *et al*. Postjunctional α-adrenoceptors in human superficial epigastric arteries and veins. Pharmacology and Toxicology 1987; 60 : 43-50.

13. Daly CJ, McGrath JC, Wilson VG. Evidence that the population of postjunctional-adrenoceptors mediating contraction of smooth muscle in the rabbit isolated ear vein is predominantly α_2. Br J Pharmacol 1988; 94 : 1085-1090.

14. Gout B. Identification and characterization of 3H-Rauwolscience binding to alpha$_2$-adrenoceptors in the canine saphenous vein. Life Sciences 1988; 43 : 1961-1971.

15. Milnor WR, Stone DN, Sastre A. Contributions of Alpha$_1$- and Alpha$_2$-adrenoceptors to contractile response in canine blood vessels. Blood Vessels 1988; 25 : 199-208.

16. Flavahan NA, Miller VM, Aarhus LL, *et al*. Denervation augments alpha-2 but not alpha-l adrenergic responses in canine saphenous veins. J Pharmacol Exper Ther 1987; 240; 589-593.

17. Komori K, Flavahan NA, Miller VM, *et al*. Electrophysiological analysis of adrenergic neurotransmission and its modulation by chronic denervation in canine saphenous veins. J Pharmacol Exper Ther 1990; 252 : 1197-1201.

18. Göthert M, Kollecker RP, Rohm N, *et al*. Inhibitory presynaptic 5-hydroxytryptamine (5-HT) receptors on the sympathetic nerves of the human saphenous vein. Naunym-Schmiedeberg's Arch Pharmacol 1986; 332 : 317-323.

19. Levitt B, Hieble JP. Prejunctional α_2-adrenoceptors modulate stimulation-evoked norepinephrine release in rabbit lateral saphenous vein. Eur J Pharmacol 1986; 132 : 197-205.

20. Benjamin N, Collier JG, Webb DJ. Angiotensin II augments sympathetically induced venoconstriction in man. Clin Sci 1988; 75 : 337-340.

21. Molderings GJ, Likungu J, Hentrich F, *et al*. Facilitatory presynaptic angiotensin receptors on the sympathetic nerves of the human saphenous vein and pulmonary artery. Potential involvement in β-adrenoceptor-mediated facilitation of noradrenaline release. Naunyn-Schmiedeberg's Arch Pharmacol 1988, 338 : 228-233.

22. Molderings G, Likungu J, Zerkowski HR, *et al.* Presynaptic β_2-adrenoceptors on the sympathetic nerve fibers of the human saphenous vein : no evidence for involvement in adrenaline-mediated positive feedback loop regulating noradrenergic transmission. Naunyn-Schmiedeberg's Arch Pharmacol 1988; 337 : 408-414.

23. Stein EZ, Trachte GJ. Thromboxane mimetics enhance adrenergic neurotransmission in the rabbit-isolated portal vein. J Cardiovasc Pharmacol 1989; 14 : 469-474.

24. Arner M, Högestätt ED. Contractile effects of noradrenaline and 5-hydroxytryptamine in human hand veins : a pharmacological receptor characterization. Acta Physiol Scand 1986; 128 : 209-217.

25. Miller VM, Komori K, Burnett JC, *et al.* Differential sensitivity to endothelin in canine arteries and veins. Am J Physiol 1989, 257 : H1127-H1131.

26. Greene AS, Shoukas AA. Changes in canine cardiac function and venous return curves by the carotid baroreflex. Am J Physiol 1986; 251 : H288-H296.

27. Hoka S, Bosnjak Z, Siker D, *et al.* Dynamic changes in venous outflow by baroreflex and left ventricular distension. Am J Physiol 1988; 254 : R212-R221.

28. Sumner A, Zelis R, Bennett M, *et al.* Effect of the venodilated state on sympathetic-induced venoconstriction in normal subjects. Am J Cardiol 1989; 63 : 973-976.

29. Vanhoutte PM, Flavahan NA. Effects of temperature on α-adrenoceptors in limb veins : role of receptor reserve. Federation Proc 1986; 45 : 2347-2354.

30. Flavahan NA, Vanhoutte PM. Thermosensitivity of cutaneous and deep veins. Phlebology 1988; 3 (Suppl 1) : 41-45.

31. Flavahan NA, Vanhoutte PM. Sympathetic purinergic vasoconstriction and therosensitivity in a canine cutaneous vein. J Pharmacol Exper Ther 1986; 239 : 784-789.

32. Hirst GDS, Jobling P. The distribution of α-adrenoceptors and P_2 purinoceptors in mesenteric arteries and veins of the guinea-pig. Br J Pharmacol 1989; 96 : 993-999.

33. Thulesius O, Ugaily-Thulesius L, Neglen P, *et al.* The role of the endothelium in the control of venous tone : studies on isolated human veins. Clin Physiol 1988; 8 : 359-366.

34. Miller VM, Vanhoutte PM. Is nitric oxide the only endothelium-derived relaxing factor in canine femoral veins ? Am J Physiol 1989; 257 : H1910-H1916.

35. Feletou M, Hoeffner U, Vanhoutte PM. Endothelium-dependent relaxing factors do not affect the smooth muscle of potal-mesenteric veins. Blood Vessels 1989; 26 : 21-32.

36. Lüscher T, Vanhoutte PM. The Endothelium : Modulator of Cardiovascular Function. CRC Press, Boca Raton 1990; pp 1-228.

37. Moser KM. Venous Thromboembolism. Am Rev Respir Dis 1990, 141 : 235-249.

38. Marcelon G, Verbeuren TJ, Lauressergues H, *et al.* Effect of *Ruscus aculeatus* on isolated canine cutaneous veins. Gen Pharmac 1983; 14 : 103-106.

39. Rubanyi G, Marcelon G, Vanhoutte PM. Effect of temperature on the responsiveness of cutaneous veins to the extract of *Ruscus aculeatus*. Gen Pharmac 1984; 15 : 431-434.

40. Harker CT, Marcelon G, Vanhoutte PM. Temperature, oestrogens and contractions of venous smooth muscle of the rabbit. Phlebology 1988; 3 (suppl. 1) : 77-82.

41. Marcelon G, Vanhoutte PM. Venotonic effect of *Ruscus* under variable temperature conditions *in vitro*. Phlebology 1988; Suppl. 1 : 51-54.

Return circulation and Norepinephrine : an update. Ed. P.M. Vanhoutte. John Libbey Eurotext, Paris © 1991, pp. 15-29.

2

Endothelial factors and regulation of vascular tone

U. Hoeffner*, P.M. Vanhoutte**

* Abt. fur Anesthesiologie, Klinikum Grosshadern,
Merchioninistr. 15, 8000 Munchen, Germany
** Center for Experimental Therapeutics, Baylor College of Medicine,
Houston, TX 77030, USA

In the last ten years, the knowledge of the physiology and pharmacology of the blood vessel wall has been considerably altered by the discovery that in isolated arteries an endothelial cell signal is required to mediate the relaxation caused by a variety of vasoactive substances *(Figure 1)* [1-5]. Furchgott and Zawadzki first reported that endothelial cells play an obligatory role in the relaxation caused by acetylcholine in isolated rabbit arteries [6]. This observation reconciled the earlier contradictory findings that acetylcholine caused dilatation in the intact organism where the endothelium is present, but contraction of most isolated blood vessels where, in most cases, the investigators had unintentionally removed the endothelial cells during the preparation. It soon became apparent that endothelial cells can also generate vasoconstrictor signals [7].

Endothelial cells represent far more than a single layer of cells that separate the blood from the tissue and at the capillary level permit the exchange of nutrients and waste products. In fact, these cells react to mechanical forces and to a number of substances, either produced locally or circulating in the blood. Their broad spectrum of metabolic activities includes the uptake and enzymatic destruction of circulating norepinephrine and 5-hydroxytryptamine (serotonin), the conversion of angiotensin I to the potent vasoconstric-

15

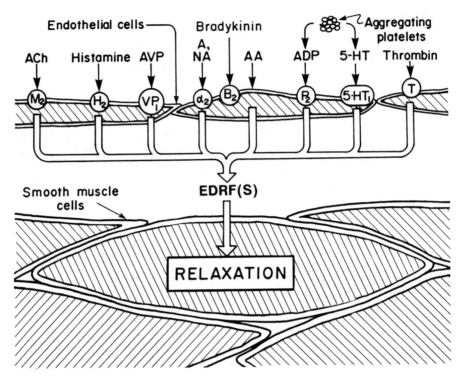

Figure 1. – Neurohumoral mediators which cause the release of endothelium-derived relaxing factor (EDRF) through activation of specific endothelial receptors (indicated by circles). In addition, EDRF can be released independent of receptor-operated mechanisms by the calcium ionophore A23187 (not shown). A=adrenaline (epinephrine), AA=arachidonic acid, Ach=acetylcholine, ADP=adenosine diphosphate, α=alpha-adrenergic receptor, AVP=arginine vasopressin, B=kininreceptor, H=histaminergic receptor, 5-HT=serotonin (5-hydroxytryptamine), serotonergic receptor, M=muscarinic receptor, NA=noradrenaline (norepinephrine), P=purinergic receptor, T=thrombin receptor, and VP=vasopressinergic receptor. (From reference 48, by permission).

tor angiotensin II and the breakdown of the potent vasodilator bradykinin into inactive peptides *(Figure 2)*. In addition, endothelial cells are the major source of prostacyclin, which can cause vasodilatation by acting directly on the vascular smooth muscle, although the main physiological function of prostacyclin probably is to prevent platelet aggregation. Indeed, in most cases, endothelium-dependent relaxations of animal and human blood vessels are not due to the production of prostacyclin, but to the production of another short-lived substance, endothelium-derived relaxing factor (EDRF) which is inactivated in the plasma, and thus, is unlikely to play a hormonal role.

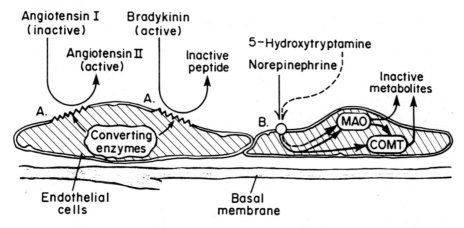

Figure 2. – The handling of bioactive substances by the pulmonary capillaries. A : Substances such as angiotensin I and bradykinin are transformed by converting enzyme located on the endothelial cell membrane, with resulting formation of active and inactive components, respectively. B : Substances such as norepinephrine and 5-hydroxytryptamine are actively taken up (o) and degraded enzymatically by monoamine oxidase (MAO) and catechol-*O*-methyltransferase (COMT). Other substances metabolically degraded by the lung include prostaglandins (not shown). (From reference 48, by permission).

Nature of endothelium-derived relaxing factors

Theoretically, cell to cell conduction could pass the signal onward from the endothelium to the smooth muscle. Electrophysiological conduction of impulses from the endothelium to the underlying vascular smooth muscle is likely to occur at the microcirculatory level, where gap junctions exist between the two type of cells - or even in larger arteries, where fenestrae in the elastic laminae allow contact between the endothelium and the deeper layers. However, in most large arteries and veins, bioassay studies have demonstrated convincingly that the endothelial cells produce a vasodilator substance, that can diffuse to the vascular smooth muscle and cause its relaxation [6, 8, 9]. This vasodilator substance is a very labile compound and under most conditions has a very short half-life, ranging from 6 to 30 seconds. It is rapidly destroyed by superoxide anions and protected by a number of antioxidant substances [9, 10].

The proposal by Furchgott [11] and Ignarro and colleagues [12] led to the demonstration that endothelial cells produce nitric oxide, the activity of

17

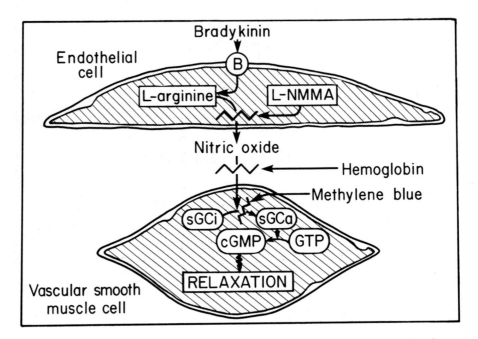

Figure 3. – Schematic representation of the production of endothelium-derived NO from L-arginine and the inhibitory effect of L-N^G-monomethyl arginine (L-NMMA). The NO derived from the endothelial cells enters the vascular smooth muscle and activates the endothelial-soluble guanylate cyclase (sGC) leading to the accumulation of cyclic guanosine monophosphate (cGMP). The schematic also shows that hemoglobin inactivates NO, while methylene blue prevents the activation of sGC ; i=inactive, a=active, and GTP=guanosine triphosphate, B=kinin-receptor.

which is indistinguishable from that of endothelium-derived relaxing factor [13]. It is very likely that the nitric oxide, enzymatically formed from L-arginine by nitric oxide synthetase in the endothelial cells, is responsible for the activation of the soluble guanylate cyclase, which, through the resultant increase in intracellular levels of cyclicGMP induces relaxation of the vascular smooth muscle *(Figure 3)* [13-16].

Nitric oxide is not the only endothelium-derived relaxing substance. Pharmacological experiments with perfused canine blood vessels indicate that another relaxing factor is released together with nitric oxide [17,18]. It causes hyperpolarization of the cell membrane, of the smooth muscle, and has been termed endothelium-derived hyperpolarizing factor (EDHF) *(Figure 4)* [19-22].

18

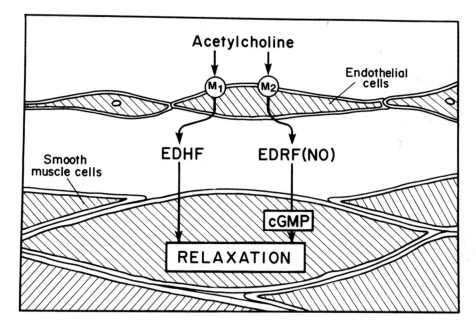

Figure 4. – The endothelial cells, when exposed to acetylcholine release two vasoactive factors. EDHF hyperpolarizes the cell membrane, thus initiating the relaxation and/or making the vascular smooth muscle more sensitive to the action of EDRF which presumably is NO. The latter sustains the relaxation by entering the cell and activating soluble guanylate cyclase which leads to an accumulation of cyclic GMP (cGMP). The muscarinic receptors (M) on the endothelial cell membrane triggering the release of the two factors do not belong to the same subtype. (From reference 48, by permission).

Physiological role

The most likely stimuli of endothelium-dependent relaxations in the intact organism are the shear stress exerted by the blood (which is responsible for flow-induced vasodilatation), locally produced autacoids such as bradykinin, histamine and substance P (which are responsible for the local hyperemia of inflammatory reactions) and the processes associated with platelet aggregation and the coagulation of blood. Thus, thrombin causes profound endothelium-dependent relaxations in a variety of isolated blood vessels including human arteries [23-25]. Platelets can induce contractions of isolated blood vessels from which the endothelium has been removed. But if endothelial cells are present, they exert a considerable braking effect on the vasoconstrictor response to the platelet products. If the blood vessels are contracted

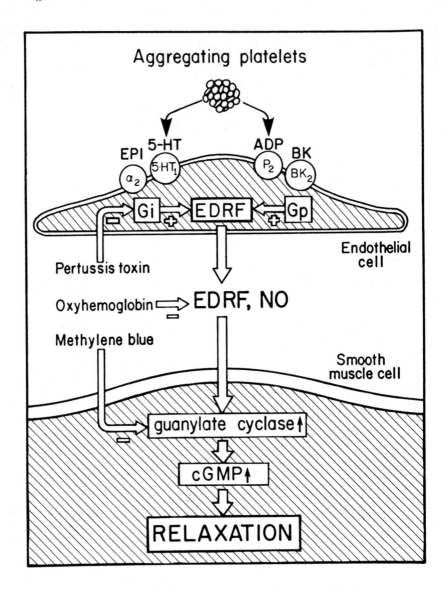

Figure 5. – The release of EDRF by endothelial cells involves at least two types of signal-transducing G-proteins, one of which is sensitive to pertussis toxin. Agonists at the endothelial cell membrane can use one and/or the other pathway. $\alpha_2 = \alpha_2$-adrenoceptor, ADP=adenosine diphosphate, BK=bradykinin, kinin receptor, cGMP=cyclic GMP, EDRF=endothelium-derived relaxing factor, Gi and Gp=G_i and G_p-proteins, 5-HT=serotonin, serotonin receptor, NO=nitric oxide, and $P_2 = P_{2y}$-purinoceptor (From reference 49, by permission).

prior to exposure to the aggregating platelets, these will cause relaxation, but only in the presence of endothelial cells. Endothelium-dependent relaxation in response to aggregating platelets is mediated by the serotonin and adenine nucleotides (ATP, ADP) that they release *(Figure 5)* [26, 27]. It is very likely

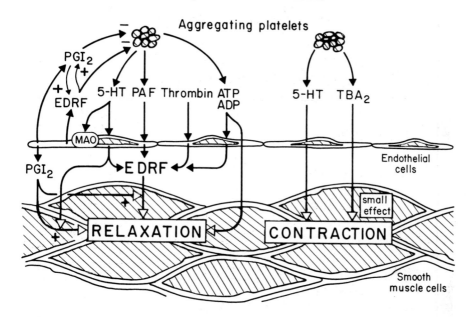

Figure 6. – Interactions between platelet products, thrombin and the endothelium. If the endothelium is intact, several of the substances released from the platelets [in particular, the adenine nucleotides (ADP and ATP) and serotonin (5-HT) and to a much lesser extent platelet activating factor (PAF)] cause the release of endothelium-derived relaxing factor (EDRF) and prostacyclin (PGI_2). The same is true for any thrombin formed. The released EDRF will relax the underlying vascular smooth muscle, opening up the blood vessel, and thus flushing the microaggregate away; it also will be released towards the lumen of the blood vessel to brake platelet adhesion to the endothelium and, synergistically with prostacyclin inhibit platelet aggregation. In addition, monoamine oxidase (MAO) and other enzymes will break down the vasoconstrictor serotonin, limiting the amount of the monoamine that can diffuse toward the smooth muscle. Finally (right) the endothelium acts as a physical barrier that prevents the access to the smooth muscle of the vasoconstrictor platelet products serotonin and thromboxane A_2 (TBA_2). These different functions of the endothelium play a key role in preventing unwanted coagulation of blood and vasospastic episodes in blood vessels with a normal intima. If the endothelial cells are removed (e.g. by trauma) the protective role of the endothelium is lost locally, platelets can adhere and aggregate and vasoconstriction follows : this contributes to the vascular phase of hemostasis, +=activation and -=inhibition. (From reference 4 by permission).

that the endothelium-dependent relaxations induced by aggregating platelets and thrombin contribute to the protective role played by the endothelium against unwanted intraluminal platelet aggregation and coagulation *(Figure 6)* [28].

Endothelium-derived contracting factors

Endothelial cells also can produce substances that cause contraction of the underlying vascular smooth muscle (endothelium-derived contracting factor(s), EDCF) [30]. The release of one of these contracting factors requires the activity of cyclooxygenase; likely candidates to explain cyclooxygenase-dependent, endothelium-dependent contractions are thromboxane A_2 and superoxide anions *(Figure 7)*. Such responses have been described in isolated canine veins and cerebral arteries [31,33] as well as in blood vessels from hypertensive animals [33]. For example, in the aorta of the spontaneously hypertensive rate, an indomethacin-sensitive contracting factor is release by acetylcholine, whereas blood vessels of normotensive rats release only relaxing factors under the same experimental conditions. The contraction evoked by the endothelial factor is mediated by stimulation of thromboxane A_2/prostaglandin H_2 receptors [34]. Once the endothelium-derived contracting factor has been released, the constrictor response predominates despite the continuous concomitant release of relaxing factor(s).

An endothelium-derived contracting peptide has been isolated by Yanagisawa and colleagues from the culture supernatant of porcine endothelial cells. This peptide, endothelin, shows homologies to a group of peptide neurotoxins that act on Na^+-channels *(Figure 8)* [35]. In certain blood vessels, the contractions evoked by endothelin are attenuated by calcium channel blockers [36]. The characteristic pattern of contraction evoked by endothelin is extremely slow in onset and long lasting [35, 37, 38]. It is uncertain whether or not endothelin contributes to the local regulation of vascular tone under physiological conditions.

In contrast to the pattern of response to endothelin, another contracting factor is released by anoxic endothelial cells, whereby the response is very rapid in onset and poorly sustained [39, 41]. The metabolism of arachidonic acid is not involved in the endothelium-dependent contraction triggered by anoxia [39-41]. The identity of the endothelium-derived contracting factor released during anoxic contraction cannot be bioassayed under conditions where for example EDRF and endothelin can be demonstrated; it is not likely to be endothelin [42].

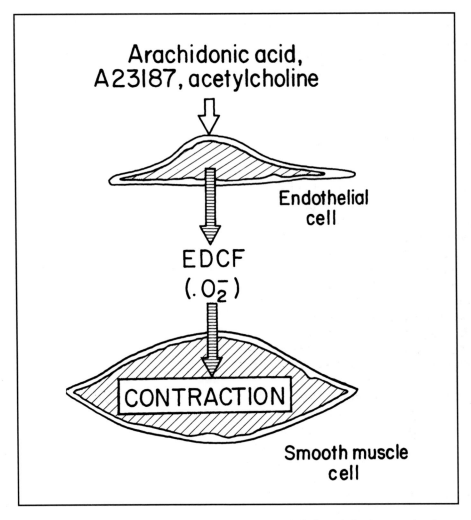

Figure 7. – Proposal that superoxide anion (O_2^-) is the endothelium-derived contracting factor (EDCF) released by arachidonic acid, the Ca^{2+} ionophore A23187 and acetylcholine from the endothelial cells of the canine basilar artery. (From reference 48, by permission).

The functional antagonism between endothelium derived contracting and relaxing factors could control locally vascular tone. Indeed, interactions between contracting and relaxing factors occur both in animal and human blood vessels [43, 44]. Under pathological conditions, the role of contracting factors may become even more important, since the release of endothelium derived relaxing factors is usually reduced. In peripheral veins, the endothe-

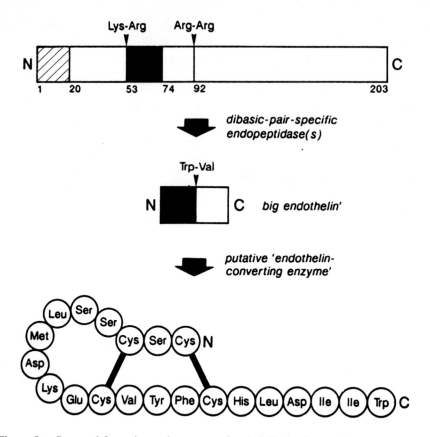

Figure 8. – Proposed formation and structure of endothelin-l. The putative secretory signal sequence (shaded box) and the endothelin sequence (black box) of the proendothelin sequence are shown. A 39-amino acid residue intermediate ("big endothelin") is generated from proendothelin by proteolytic cleavage at paired basic residues. The final 21-amino acid product endothelin-l finally is cleaved from big endothelin by a putative converting enzyme. C=carboxy terminal, N=nitrogenterminal of the peptide. (From reference 35, by permission) .

lium appears to release relatively little EDRF, while endothelium-dependent contractions are prominent [7].

Clinical importance

Internal mammary arteries and saphenous veins are both used as bypass grafts in patients with coronary artery disease [45]. Internal mammary arteries exhibit a much larger endothelium-dependent response to acetylcholine than the saphenous veins *(Figure 9)* [44]. This difference persists when comparing arterial and venous grafts supplying the same vascular bed. Different biological properties of the arteries and veins, specially the arterial and venous endothelium, may cause the higher potency of arterial grafts compared to venous grafts. The more effective release of endothelium derived relaxing factor in the arteries may allow them to adapt more effectively to the flow requirement of the coronary circulation than the veins.

As mentioned earlier, the release of endothelium dependent relaxing factors in response mainly to thrombin and ADP may provide an important protective mechanism against platelet induced thrombus formation, since at sites where platelets are activated the local blood flow would increase and flush away and desegregate any evolving platelet clot [46, 47]. Furthermore, an intact endothelium is the major source of prostacyclin production, which

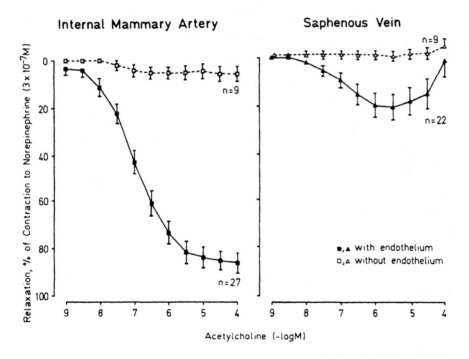

Figure 9. – Effects of acetylcholine in the isolated human internal mammary artery (left) and saphenous vein (right). The muscarinic agonist evokes relaxations in preparations with (solid symbols), but not in those without endothelium (open symbols). Endothelium-dependent relaxations are more pronounced in the arteries than in the veins. (From reference 45, by permission).

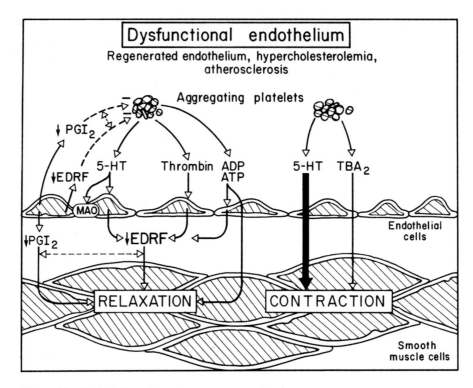

Figure 10. – Endothelium-dependent responses under pathologic conditions. The endothelium is dysfunctional in the regenerated state, hypercholesterolemia, and atherosclerosis, releasing less endothelium-derived relaxing factor (EDRF), while the ability of the smooth muscle to contract is unaltered. As a result, the contractions predominate. In atherosclerosis, the production of both endothelium-dependent relaxing factor and prostacyclin (PGI_2) is reduced, and their synergistic actions against aggregating platelets may not occur. ADP=adenosine diphosphate, ATP=adenosine triphosphate, 5-HT=serotonin, MAO=monamine oxidase, TBA_2=thromboxane A_2,-=inhibition, and +=synergism. (From reference 50, with permission of the American Heart Association).

causes further vasodilatation. Endothelium-dependent relaxation in response to aggregating platelets are reduced chronically after trauma, when the endothelial cells have regenerated [29]. An abnormal function of the endothelium may facilitate the occurrence of vasospastic episodes in response to the platelet products, particularly in coronary arteries [27, 29]. Under physiological conditions, the absence of endothelium permits the vascular phase of hemostasis. Under pathological circumstances, the absence or dysfunction of the endothelium favors the occurrence of abnormal platelet adhesion and aggregation with resulting release not only of vasoconstrictors such as serotonin and thromboxane A_2 (that favor vasospasm), but also of growth factors (that favor morphological alterations of the blood vessel wall) *(Figure 10).* Thus the dysfunction of the endothelium in terms of the release of relaxing and contracting factors could greatly contribute to the abnormalities observed in hypertensive and atherosclerotic blood vessels [4, 48].

References

1. Furchgott RF. Role of the endothelium in responses of vascular smooth muscle. Circ Res 1983; 53 : 557-573.

2. Peach MJ, Loeb AL, Singer HA, *et al.* Endothelium-derived vascular relaxing factor. Hypertension 1985; 7 (Suppl 1) : 94-100.

3. Vanhoutte PM, Rubanyi GM, Miller VM, *et al.* Modulation of vascular smooth muscle contraction by the endothelium. Annu Rev Physiol 1986; 48 : 307-320.

4. Vanhoutte PM. The endothelium : modulator of vascular smooth muscle tone. N Engl J Med 1988; 319 : 512-513.

5. Bassenge E, Busse R. Endothelial modulation of coronary tone. Prog Cardiol Dis 1987; 30 : 349-380.

6. Furchgott RF, Zawadzki JV. The obligatory role of endothelial cells in the relaxation of arterial smoth muscle by acetylcholine. Nature 1980; 299 : 373-376.

7. DeMey JG, Vanhoutte PM. Heterogeneous behavior of the canine arterial and venous wall : importance of the endothelium. Circ Res 1982; 51 : 439-447.

8. Griffith TM, Henderson AH, Edwards DH, *et al.* Isolated perfused rabbit coronary artery and aortic strip preparations : the role of endothelium-derived relaxant factor. J Physiol 1984; 351 : 13-24.

9. Rubanyi GM, Lorenz RR, Vanhoutte PM. Bioassay of endothelium-derived relaxing factor(s) : inactivation by catecholamines. Am J Physiol 1985; 249 : H95-H101.

10. Rubanyi GM, Vanhoutte PM. Superoxide anions and hyperoxia inactivate endothelium-derived relaxing factor. Am J Physiol 1986; 250 : H822-H827.

11. Furchgott RF. Studies on relaxation of rabbit aorta by sodium nitrite : the basis for the proposal that acid-activatable inhibitory factor from bovine retractor penis is inorganic nitrite and the endothelium-derived relaxing factor is nitric oxide, *In:Vasodilation:Vascular Smooth Muscle, Peptides, Autonomic Nerves and Endothelium,* Vanhoutte PM, Ed., Raven Press, New York, 1988; 401-414.

12. Ignarro LJ, Byrns RE, Buga GM, *et al.* Endothelium-derived relaxing factor from pulmonary artery and vein possesses pharmacological and chemical properties identical to those of nitric oxide radical. Circ Res 1987; 61 : 866-879.

13. Holzmann S. Endothelium-induced relaxation by acetylcholine associated with large rises in cyclic GMP in coronary arterial strips. J Cyclic Nucleot Res 1982; 8 : 409-419.

14. Ignarro LJ, Byrns RE, Wood KS. Endothelium-dependent modulation of cGMP levels and intrinsic smooth muscle tone in isolated bovine intrapulmonary artery and vein. Circ Res 1987; 60 : 82-92.

15. Förstermann U, Mülsch A, Böhme E, *et al.* Stimulation of soluble guanylate cyclase by an acetylcholine-induced endothelium-derived factor from rabbit and canine arteries. Circ Res 1986; 58 : 531-538.

16. Rapoport RM, Murad F. Agonist-induced endothelium-dependent relaxation in rat thoracic aorta may be mediated through cGMP. Circ Res 1983; 52 : 352-357.

17. Vanhoutte PM. The end of the quest ? Nature 1987; 327 : 459-460.

18. Hoeffner U, Feletou M, Flavahan NA, *et al.* Canine arteries release two different endothelium-derived relaxing factors. Am J Physiol 1989; 257 : H330-H333.

19. Bolton TB, Clapp LH. Endothelial-dependent relaxant actions of carbachol and substance P in arterial smooth muscle. Br J Pharmacol 1986; 87 : 713-723.

20. Feletou M, Vanhoutte PM. Endothelium-dependent hyperpolarization of canine coronary smooth muscle. Br. J Pharmacol 1988; 93 : 515-524.

21. Alonso MY, Salaries M, Barris MT, *et al.* Endothelial factors released by acetylcholine in cat cerebral and femoral arteries. Archives Inter de Pharmaco et de Ther 1990, 305, 226.

22. Komori K, Suzuki H. Electrical responses of smooth muscle cells during cholinergic vasodilation in the rabbit saphenous artery. Circ Res 1987; 61 : 586-593.

23. Lüscher TF, Cooke JP, Houston DS, *et al.,* Endothelium-dependent relaxations in human peripheral and renal arteries. Mayo Clin Proc 1987; 62 : 601-606.

24. Vanhoutte PM, Miller VM. Heterogeneity of endothelium-dependent responses in mammalian blood vessels. J Cardiovasc Pharmacol 1985; 7 (Suppl 3) : 512-523.

25. Katusic ZS, Shepherd JT, Vanhoutte PM. Oxytocin causes endothelium-dependent relaxations of canine basilar arteries by activating V1-vasopressinergic receptors. J Pharmacol Exp Ther 1986; 236 : 166-170,.

26. Cohen RA, Shepherd JT, Vanhoutte PM. Inhibitory role of the endothelium in the response of isolated coronary arteries to platelets. Science 1983; 221 : 273-274.

27. Houston DS, Shepherd JT, Vanhoutte PM. Aggregating human platelets cause direct contraction and endothelium-dependent relaxation in isolated canine coronary arteries. J Clin Invest 1986; 78 : 539-544.

28. Vanhoutte PM, Houston DS. Platelets, endothelium and vasopasm. Circulation 1985 ; 72 : 728-734.

29. Shimokawa H, Aarhus LL, Vanhoutte PM. Porcine coronary arteries with regenerated endothelium have a reduced endothelium-dependent responsiveness to aggregating platelets and serotonin. Circ Res 1987; 61 : 256-270.

30. Vanhoutte PM. Endothelium-dependent contractions in arteries and veins. Blood Vessels 1987; 24 : 141-144.

31. Miller VM, Vanhoutte PM. Endothelium-dependent contractions to arachidonic acid are mediated by products of cyclooxygenase in canine veins. Am J Physiol 1985; 248 : H432-H437.

32. Katusic ZS, Shepherd JT, Vanhoutte PM. Endothelium-dependent contractions to stretch in canine basilar arteries. Am J Physiol 1987; 252 : H671-H673.

33. Lüscher T, Vanhoutte PM. Endothelium-dependent contractions to acetylcholine in the aorta of the spontaneously hypertensive rat. Hypertension 1986, 8 : 344-348.

34. Auch-Schwelk W, Katusic ZS, Vanhoutte PM. Pharmacology of endothelium-dependent contractions to acetylcholine in the SHR aorta. Arch Inter de Pharmaco et de Ther 1990; 305 : 228.

35 . Yanagisawa M, Kurihara H, Kimura S, *et al.* A novel potent vasoconstrictor peptide produced by vascular endothelial cells. Nature 1988; 332 : 411-415.

36. Igarashi Y, Aicawa ZY, Tamura M, *et al.* Vasoconstriction of endothelin on the canine coronary artery : Is a novel endogenous peptide involved in regulating myocardial blood flow and coronary spasm. Am. Heart J. 1989, 118, 674-678.

37. Hickey KA, Rubanyi GM, Paul RJ, *et al.* Characterization of a coronary vasoconstrictor produced by cultured endothelial cells. Am J Physiol 1985; 248 : C550-C556.

38. Gillespie MN, Owasoyo JO, McMurtry IF, *et al.* Sustained coronary vasoconstriction provoked by a peptidergic substance released from endothelial cells in culture. J Pharmacol Exp Ther 1986; 236 : 339-343.

39. De May JG, Vanhoutte PM. Anoxia and endothelium-dependent reactivity in canine femoral artery. J Physiol (London) 1983; 355 : 65-74.

40. Rubanyi GM, Vanhoutte PM. Hypoxia releases a vasoconstrictor substance from the canine vascular endothelium. J Physiol (London) 1985; 364 : 45-56.

41. Katusic ZS, Shepherd JT, Vanhoutte PM. Anoxic contractions in isolated cerebral arteries. Contribution of endothelium-derived factors, metabolites of arachidonic acid and calcium entry. J Cardiovasc Pharmacol 1986; 8(Suppl 8) : 97-101.

42. Vanhoutte PM, Auch-Schwelk W, Boulanger C, *et al.* Does endothelin-1 mediate endothelium-dependent contractions during anoxia ? J Cardiovasc Pharmacol 1989 ; 13 (Suppl 5) : 124-128.

43. Lüscher TF, Vanhoutte PM. Endothelium-dependent responses in human blood vessels. Trends Pharm Sci 1988; 9 : 181-184.

44. Lüscher TF, Yang Z, Diederich D, *et al.* Endothelium-derived vasoactive substances : Potential role in hypertension and atherosclerosis and vascular occlusion. J Cardiovasc Pharmacol 1989; 14 (Suppl 6) : 63-69.

45. Lüscher TF, Diederich D, Siebenmann R, *et al.* Differences between endothelium-dependent relaxations in arterial and in venous coronary bypass grafts. N Engl J Med 1988 ; 319 : 462-467.

46. Lüscher TF. *In:Endotelial Vasoactive Substances and Cardiovascular Disease.* S Karger Basel, 1988, 1-133.

47. Förstermann U, Mügge A, Bode SM, *et al.* Response of human coronary arteries to aggregating platelets : Importance of endothelium-derived relaxing factor and prostanoids. Circ Res 1988; 63 : 306-312.

48. Lüscher T, Vanhoutte PM. The Endothelium : Modulator of Cardiovascular Function. CRC Press, Boca Raton, Florida, 1990; 1-228.

49. Vanhoutte PM. Endothelium-derived vasoactive factors. Hypertension Annual, in press.

50. Vanhoutte PM, Shimokawa H. Endothelium-derived relaxing factor(s) and coronary vasospasm. Circulation 1989; 80 No. 1 : 1-9.

Return circulation and Norepinephrine : an update. Ed. P.M. Vanhoutte. John Libbey Eurotext, Paris © 1991, pp. 31-42.

3

Ruscus extract releases endothelium-derived relaxing factor in arteries and veins

V.M. Miller*, G. Marcelon**, P.M. Vanhoutte***

* Department of Physiology, Mayo Clinic and Foundation,
Rochester, MN 55905, USA
** Centre de Recherches Pierre Fabre, 17, avenue Jean-Moulin,
Castres 81106, France
*** Center for Experimental Therapeutics, Baylor College of Medicine,
Houston, TX 77030, USA

Introduction

The extract of *Ruscus aculeatus* is used to treat venous insufficiency which is often associated with pregnancy and premenstrual syndrome [1,2]. The extract is a venoconstrictor that stimulates both $alpha_1$ and $alpha_2$-adrenoceptors on vascular smooth muscle and displaces endogenous norepinephrine from adrenergic nerve endings [3, 4]. Endothelial cells of canine arteries are endowed with $alpha_2$-adrenoceptors which are linked to the release of endothelium-derived relaxing factor [5-7]. Endothelium-dependent responses depend on the hormonal states of the animal [8-10]. Experiments were designed to determine whether or not *Ruscus*-extract could stimulate the endothelial cells of arteries and veins to release vasoactive factors and if so whether such a response could be modulated by the hormonal state of the animal.

Methods

Animal model

Adult female mongrel dogs (15-20kg) were anesthetized with sodium pentobarbital (30 mg/kg, intravenously) and the ovaries were removed through a midline abdominal incision using aseptic surgical techniques. At the time of surgery, pellets (Innovative Research of America, Toledo, Ohio) containing either a carrier substance, 17β-estradiol (estrogen ; 35 mg/pellet/dog), progesterone (250 mg/pellet; 8 pellets/dog), or a combination of estrogen (1 pellet/dog) plus progesterone (8 pellets/dog) were implanted subcutaneously.

In vitro experiments

After 16-25 days, the dogs again were anesthetized and arterial blood samples were obtained for the determination of serum levels of hormones. The animals were exsanguinated through the carotid arteries and the left circumflex coronary artery and femoral vein were removed. The blood vessels were cleaned of connective tissue and cut into rings. In some rings, the endothelium was removed by gently rubbing the intimal surface with a cotton swab. Rings with and without endothelium were suspended for the measurement of isometric force in organ chambers filled with aerated (95 % O_2-5 % CO_2) modified Krebs-Ringer bicarbonate solution (control solution ; millimolar composition : NaCl, 118.3 ; KCl, 4.7 ; $CaCl_2$, 2.5 ; $MgSO_4$, 1.2 ; KH_2PO_4, 1.2; $NaHCO_3$, 25.0; calcium disodium edetate, 0.026; and glucose, 11.1).

Each ring was stretched to the optimal point on its length-tension curve as determined by the tension developed to KCl (20mM) or norepinephrine (3×10^{-7}M). The presence of the endothelium was determined by the absence or presence of relaxations to acetylcholine (3×10^{-7}M) during contraction to prostaglandin $F_{2\alpha}$ (2×10^{-6}M ; coronary arteries) or norepinephrine (3×10^{-7}M; femoral veins). The coronary arteries were incubated with indomethacin (10^{-5}M) and the femoral veins with indomethacin plus propranolol (5×10^{-6}M) for 40 minutes. Cumulative concentration-response curves to *Ruscus*-extract (10^{-6} to 10^{-3}g/ml) were obtained either under basal conditions (veins) or during contractions to prostaglandin $F_{2\alpha}$ (2×10^{-6}M; coronary arteries) or norepinephrine (3×10^{-7}M; femoral veins). In some experiments, the rings were incubated with methylene blue (10^{-5}M for 30 minutes) or hemoglobin (10^{-5}M for five minutes) before and during the response to *Ruscus*-extract.

Drugs and chemicals

The following drugs (all from Sigma Chemical Co., St. Louis, MO) were used : acetylcholine chloride, adenosine diphosphate, atropine sulfate, hemoglobin (bovine), indomethacin and methylene blue. Indomethacin was dissolved in a solution of Na_2CO_3 (final bath concentration : $2x10^{-5}M$). *Ruscus aculeatus*-extract (*Ruscus ;* Pierre Fabre, Castres, France) was dissolved in dimethyl sulfoxide (final bath concentration : $1.1x10^{-1}M$). Hemoglobin was prepared by the method of Martin, *et al.* [11]. All drugs were made fresh daily and except for the *Ruscus*-extract were kept on ice until used. The concentrations of drugs are expressed as the final concentrations in the organ chamber [molar (M) or g/ml].

Calculations and statistical analysis

The results are expressed as means $\pm$ SEM. In all experiments, n equals the number of rings taken from different dogs. Where appropriate, the effective concentration causing 50 % of the maximal response (ED_{50}) was calculated for individual concentration-response curves and the mean of these values reported as the negative logarithm of the concentration. Since rings with and without endothelium of the same blood vessels were studied in parallel, Student's t-test for paired observations was used. Analysis of variance was used to compare more than two means or responses from different treatment groups. When a significant F value was obtained, a Scheffe's test was used to identify differences among means. Values were considered to be statistically different when P was less than 0.05.

Results

Serum levels of estrogen averaged about 30 ng/l00 ml in estrogen and estrogen plus progesterone-treated groups; serum levels of progesterone averaged about 400 ng/l00 ml, 750 ng/l00 ml and 2300 ng/100 ml in the estrogen, progesterone and estrogen plus progesterone-treated groups, respectively. Serum levels of both estrogen and progesterone were significantly lower in the untreated-group than in the groups with the hormonal implants.

Coronary arteries

In coronary arteries contracted with prostaglandin $F_{2\alpha}$, *Ruscus* caused concentration-dependent (3×10^{-6} to 3×10^{-4}M) decreases in tension in rings with but not without endothelium *(Figure 1)*. These relaxations were not altered significantly by the hormonal status of the animal (data not shown). The relaxations in rings with endothelium were inhibited significantly by the muscarinic antagonist, atropine (10^{-6}M), *(Figure 2)*. The inhibitor of the endothelium-derived nitric oxide, hemoglobin (10^{-5}M), and the inhibitor of soluble guanylate cyclase, methylene blue (10^{-5}M), both significantly reduced the relaxations to *Ruscus (Figures 3 et 4)*.

Femoral veins

In the femoral veins, *Ruscus* caused concentration-dependent increases in tension which were less in rings with than in those without endothelium *(Figure 5)*. Rings of veins without endothelium from estrogen plus progeste-

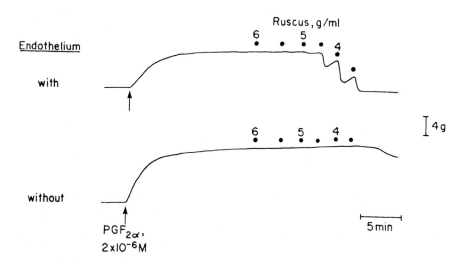

Figure 1. – Tracing of relaxations to *Ruscus* in canine coronary arteries with and without endothelium. The extract reversed the contractions to prostaglandin $F_{2\alpha}$ only in rings with endothelium. Similar results were found in 23 other experiments. All experiments were conducted in the presence of indomethacin (10^{-5}M).

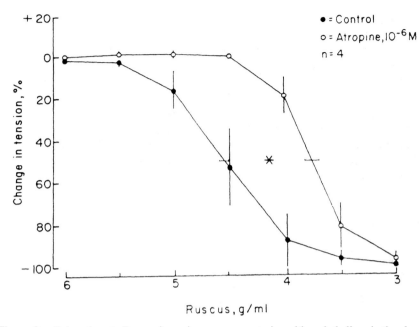

Figure 2. – Relaxations to Ruscus in canine coronary arteries with endothelium in the absence and presence of atropine (10^{-6}M). Values are expressed as a percent decrease in tension from a contraction to prostaglandin $F_{2\alpha}$ (2×10^{-6}M; 11.1 ± 1.7 and 10.8 ± 1.7, n=4, in the absence and presence of atropine, respectively). Data are shown as means $\pm$ SEM. Asterisk denotes significant difference in the concentration causing 50 % relaxation (ED_{50}) by Student's t-test for paired observations, ($P < 0.05$).

rone-treated dogs were more sensitive to the contractile effects of *Ruscus* than those from dogs treated with progesterone alone *(Figure 6),* (ED_{50} (-log g/ml) : 3.7 ± 0.1, n=7, in progesterone-treated dogs and 4.2 ± 0.2, n=5, in estrogen plus progesterone-treated dogs, $P < 0.05$).

When rings of femoral vein with endothelium were contracted with norepinephrine (3×10^{-7}M), Ruscus caused concentration-dependent relaxations. Rings from estrogen plus progesterone-treated dogs tended to be less sensitive to the inhibitory effects of the extract than those from dogs treated with progesterone alone *(Figure 7).* In rings with endothelium, relaxations to acetylcholine (3×10^{-7}M) tended to be less in estrogen plus progesterone treated dogs than in those treated with estrogen alone ($29.2 \pm 5.3\%$, n=6, and $55.8 \pm 14.9\%$, n=5, respectively, of the contraction to norepinephrine; $P < 0.05$, analysis of variance).

35

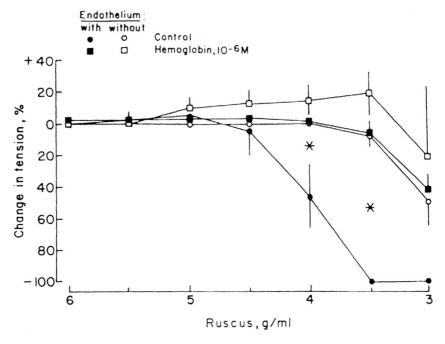

Figure 3. – Responses to Ruscus in canine coronary arteries in the absence and presence of hemoglobin (10^{-5}M). Values are expressed as a percent decrease in tension from a contraction to prostaglandin $F_{2\alpha}$ (2×10^{-6}M; 13.9 ± 1.0 g, n=3, in rings with endothelium in the absence of hemoglobin.) Neither removal of the endothelium or the presence of the hemoglobin significantly altered the contractions to prostaglandin $F_{2\alpha}$. Data are shown as means $\pm$ SEM. Asterisk denotes significant difference from rings with endothelium by Student's t-test for paired observations, ($P<0.05$).

Discussion

The present results indicate that the extract from *Ruscus* can initiate the release of vasoactive factor(s) from the endothelium of arteries and veins. The action of the endothelium-derived factors are inhibitory to contractions initiated by the extract itself, by prostaglandin $F_{2\alpha}$ and by norepinephrine. The finding that the relaxations initiated by the extract can be inhibited by atropine suggests, at least in arteries, that the release of endothelium-derived factor(s) is mediated through stimulation of muscarinic receptors [12]. The re-

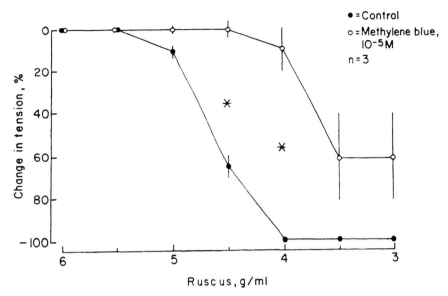

Figure 4. – Responses to *Ruscus* in canine coronary arteries with endothelium in the absence and presence of methylene blue (10^{-5}M). Values are expressed as a percent decrease in tension from a contraction to prostaglandin $F_{2\alpha}$ (2×10^{-6}M; 5.8 ± 1.9 g and 9.5 ± 1.3, n=3, in rings with endothelium in the absence and presence of methylene blue, respectively.) Data are shown as means $\pm$ SEM. Asterisk denotes significant difference by Student's t-test for paired observations, ($P < 0.05$).

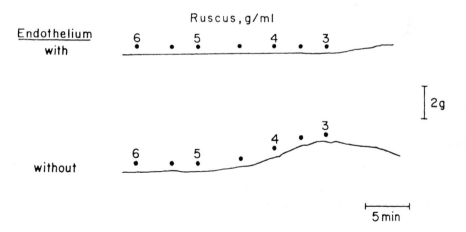

Figure 5. – Tracing of the responses to *Ruscus* in femoral veins with (top) and without (bottom) endothelium from an ovariectomized dog. Experiments were conducted in the presence of indomethacin (10^{-5}M) and propranolol (5×10^{-6}M). Similar results were obtained in four other experiments in ovariectomized dogs treated with hormones.

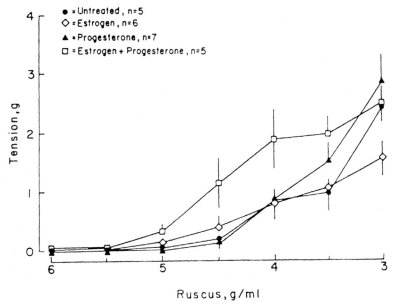

Figure 6. Contractions to *Ruscus* in canine femoral veins without endothelium. Experiments were conducted in the presence of indomethacin (10^{-5}M) and propranolol (5×10^{-6}M). Data are shown as means ± SEM of the grams of tension developed to the extract.

laxing factor released by *Ruscus* in the present studies probably is not prostacylin as all experiments were carried out in the presence of indomethacin which inhibits the metabolism of arachidonic acid by cylooxygenase.

In the coronary arteries, the relaxing factor(s) released by the extract shares some chemical characteristics with nitric oxide. This conclusion is based on the observations that the relaxations are inhibited by hemoglobin which inactivates nitric oxide [11-14] and by methylene blue which inhibits soluble guanylate cyclase [11, 15]. Increases in cyclic guanosine monophosphate (cyclic GMP) mediate the relaxations to nitric oxide in arterial smooth muscle [16, 17].

The venoconstrictor effects of the *Ruscus* extract are influenced not only by the integrity of the endothelial cells but also by the hormonal state of the animal. This conclusion is supported by the observations that contractions to the extract are greater in veins without endothelium and that veins from dogs treated with a combination of estrogen plus progesterone were more sensitive to the excitatory effects of *Ruscus* than veins from the other hormone-treated groups.

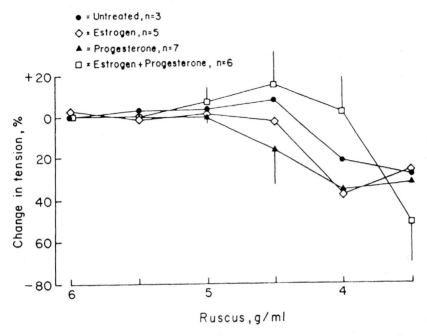

Figure 7. – Responses to *Ruscus* in canine femoral veins with endothelium. Experiments were conducted in the presence of indomethacin (10^{-5}M) and propranolol (5×10^{-6}M). Values are shown as percent change in tension from a contraction to norepinephrine (3×10^{-7}M) which did not differ among treatment groups (pooled value = 3.4 ± 4 g, n=18). Data are expressed as means; for clarity, standard errors are omitted for the responses of the untreated- and estrogen-treated groups.

The reasons that the endothelium-dependent relaxations to *Ruscus* tended to be less prominent in veins from the estrogen plus progesterone treated-group are not clear. It may represent a direct effect of the hormone-treatment on the ability of the endothelial cells to produce relaxing factor because in the veins the relaxations initiated by acetylcholine also tended to be less pronounced in the presence of estrogen plus progesterone. Alternatively, when serum levels of estrogen and progesterone are elevated, the increased sensitivity of the smooth muscle to the contractile components of the extract may reduce the ability of the veins to be inhibited by endothelium-derived relaxing factors which act as functional antagonists to the contraction [18]. The distribution of receptors and their coupling to the production and release of endothelium-derived factor may be dissimilar between arteries and veins, as the endothelium-dependent relaxations to *Ruscus* were not influenced by the hormonal treatment in arteries.

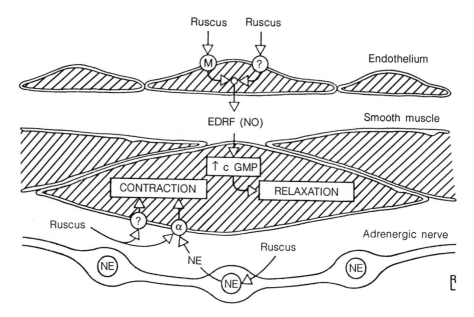

Figure 8. – Schematic showing the possible effects of *Ruscus* on the elements of the blood vessel wall. Abbreviations : α, alpha adrenergic receptor; cGMP, cyclic guanosine monophosphate; M, muscarinic receptor; NE, norepinephrine; N0, nitric oxide.

Conclusion

Components of the extract derived from *Ruscus aculeatus* now have been shown to stimulate all tissue elements of the blood vessel wall : the adrenergic nerve endings [3], the smooth muscle [3, 4] and the endothelium (present study; *Figure 8*). The stimulation of the endothelium by the extract tends to inhibit the contractions that it causes as well as to contractions caused by norepinephrine and prostaglandin $F_{2\alpha}$. Therefore, in circumstances where the endothelium may be dysfunctional, as might occur in venous varicosities [19], localized, excitatory effects of the extract would prevail. These excitatory effects may be more prominent when estrogen and progesterone are elevated as would be found during some phases of the menstrual cycle, pregnancy, and under hormonal contraceptive-treatment.

References

1. Monteil-Seurin J. Value of *Ruscus* in Gyneacological pathology-25 years fo use in private practice. Phlebology 1988 3 (1) : 87-98.
2. Cappelli R, Nicora M, Diperri T. Use of extract of *Ruscus aculeatus* in venous disease in the lower limbs. Drugs Exptl, Clin Res 1988; 14 (4) : 227-283.
3. Marcelon G, Verbeuren TJ, Lauressergues H, Vanhoutte PM. Effect of *Ruscus aculeatus* on isolated canine cutaneous veins. Gen Pharmacol 1983, 14 : 103-106.
4. Rubanyi G, Marcelon G, Vanhoutte PM. Effect of temperature on the responsiveness of cutaneous veins to the extract of *Ruscus aculeatus*. Gen Pharmacol 1984; 15 : 431-434.
5. Cocks TM, Angus JA. Endothelium-dependent relaxation of coronary arteries by noradrenalin and serotonin. Nature 1983; 305 : 627-630.
6. Miller VM, Vanhoutte PM. Endothelial α2 adrenoceptors in canine pulmonary and systemic blood vessels. European J Pharmacol 1985; 118 : 123-129.
7. Flavahan NA, Shimokawa H, Vanhoutte PM. Pertussis toxin inhibits endothelium-dependent relaxations to certain agonists in porcine coronary arteries. J Physiol 1988; 408 : 549-560.
8. Gisclard V, Miller VM, Vanhoutte PM. Effect of 17β-estradiol on endothelium-dependent responses in the rabbit. J Pharmacol Exp Ther 1988; 244 : 19-22.
9. Miller VM, Aarhus LL, Vanhoutte PM. Effects of estrogens on adrenergic and endothelium-dependent responses in the ovarian artery of the rabbit. *In:Proceedings of the Second International Symposium on Resistance Arteries*. W Halpern, J Brayden, M McLaughlin, G Osol, BL Pegram, and K Mackey, editors. Perinatology Press, Ithaca, NY 1988; 136-145.
10. Miller VM, Vanhoutte PM. 17β-Estradiol augments endothelium-dependent contractions to arachidonic acid in rabbit aorta. Am J Physiol 1990; (in press).
11. Martin W, Villani GM, Jothianandan D, *et al.* Selective blockade of endothelium-dependent and glyceryl trinitrate-induced relaxation by hemoglobin and by methylene blue in the rabbit aorta. J Pharmacol Exp Ther 1985; 232 (3) : 708-716.
12. Furchgott RF, Zawadzki JV. The obligatory role of endothelial cells in the relaxation of arterial smooth muscle by acetylcholine. Nature 1980; 288 : 373-376.
13. Furchgott RF. Studies on relaxation of rabbit aorta by sodium nitrite : The basis for the proposal that the acid-activatable inhibitory factor from bovine retractor penis is inorganic nitrite and the endothelium-derived relaxing factor is nitric oxide. *In:Vasodilatation*. PM Vanhoutte, editor. Raven Press, New York, 1988; 401-414.
14. Ignarro LJ, Buga GM, Wood KS, *et al.* Endothelium-derived relaxing factor produced and released from artery and vein is nitric oxide. Proc Natl Acad Sci; 1987; 84 : 9265-9269.
15. Gruetter CA, Gruetter DY, Lyon JE, *et al.* Relationship between cyclic guanosine 3' : 5'-monophosphate formation and relaxation of coronary arterial smooth muscle by glyceryl trinitrate, nitroprusside, nitrite and nitric oxide : effects of methylene blue and methemoglobin. J Pharmacol Exp Ther 1981; 219 : 181-186.
16. Ignarro LJ, Byrns RE, Wood KS. Endothelium-dependent modulation of cGMP levels and intrinsic smooth muscle tone in isolated bovine intrapulmonary artery and vein. Circ Res 1987; 60 : 82-92.
17. Rapoport RM, Murad F. Agonist-induced endothelium-dependent relaxation in rat thoracic aorta may be mediated through cGMP. Circ Res 1983; 52 : 352-357.

18. Flavahan NA, Vanhoutte PM. Receptor-reserve and heterogeneity of vascular responses to vasodilator stimuli. *In:Mechanisms of Vasodilitation.* PM Vanhoutte, editor. Raven Press, New York, 1988; 201-210.
19. Bouissou H, Julian M, Pieraggi MTh, *et al.* Vein morphology Phlebology 1988; 3 (1) : 1-11.

Return circulation and Norepinephrine : an update. Ed. P.M. Vanhoutte. John Libbey Eurotext, Paris © 1991, pp. 43-53.

4

Efficacy of *Ruscus* extract* in the treatment of the premenstrual syndrome

J. Monteil-Seurin*, Ph. Ladure**

* 2, rue Richer de Belleval, 34000 Montpellier
** Centre de Recherches Pierre Fabre, 17 avenue Jean Moulin,
81106 Castres, France

The importance of the premenstrual syndrome study had been established by Franck, in 1931 [1].

Its frequency, although most differently assessed according to the studies, is considerable : Pariser [2] estimates it at 50 %, with 38 % of women suffering every month from premenstrual syndrome. This explains the social and economical disturbances it creates, in particular absenteeism. However, its consequences on the family, and on quality of life of the women themselves is hard to evaluate.

The symptomatology is polymorphous. The original symptoms described by Franck [1] have been expanded to a list of more than 50 complaints [4]. They include irritableness (Franck's " Hair trigger temper " [1]), temporary alienation, moderate weight gain, orthostatic idiopathic edema, tension in the breasts which can become unbearable mammary pain [1, 4-7]. As a consequence premenstrual syndrome takes an almost personal form for every woman [7].

---

* Cyclo-3 Fort®

Hence a definition of the premenstrual syndrome remains vague : a set of polysymptomatic psychological and/or physical manifestations occuring electively and regularly before menses. The limits between disabling and acceptable symptoms are difficult to define. The most frequently encountered symptoms can be summarized as follows :

Congestive phenomena : these concern the whole abdominal-pelvic area and include mammary tension, heaviness of the lower limbs and congestion of all mucous membranes.

Edema : infiltration occur in the skin, the subcutaneous tissue, the deep dermis, the interstitial spaces and the skeletal muscles. It prevails at the members' roots, the pelvic girdle, the abdomen and the breasts. The water retention occurs with a decrease in circulating blood volume.

Neuropsychic disturbances : bitemporal or bifrontal headaches, catamenial hemicrania, vertigo, lipothymia, psychogenic disturbances. These are the most serious symptoms of the premenstrual syndrome [8].

The physiopathology of the premenstrual syndrome is still unclear. Several mechanisms have been proposed. The premenstrual syndrome occurs during ovulatory cycles, and results from an imbalance between estrogens and progesterone. The biological control of ovulation is necessary to get rid of premenstrual syndrome disturbance [9]. Since women taking oral contraceptives do not stop complaining, Muse [10] has performed a medical ovariotomy with an LH-RH antagonist, while Hamarbäck *et al.* [11] did it with a Gn-RH antagonist : the results are rather good, although not permanent, at the cost of considerable side effect. Lagrue *et al.* [12] studying the effects of progesterone on the capillary permeability conclude in favor of the pathogenic polymorphism of the disease.

Other neuroendocrinian disturbances have been referred to : the circadian profiles of plasmatic prolactin, growth hormones and cortisol have been studied by Steiner *et al.* [13]. These authors did not find any correlation between hormonal secretory profiles and the premenstrual syndrome. The latter cannot be regarded as a psychoendocrinian model of deep depression [14].

The efficacy of vitamin B6, of magnesium, of bromocriptine or danasol, has not been verified by any serious study. The nutritional theory [15] is still to be proven right.

The aberrant release of β-endorphins causes a series of endocrinian disturbances which can result in premenstrual syndrome [16]. It is well known that an insufficiency in endorphins involves a catecholaminergic hyperactivity. Cathecholamines are the basis of the homeostatic control of venous function [17].

The notion of interaction between ovarian steroids and neurotransmitters, serotoninergic and adrenergic receptors, different peptides (opioids, vasopressin, ocytocin) is interesting. Reid and Yen [3] have insisted upon the role played by cathecholamines and opioid substances, the regulation of endorphins and enkephalins through sexual steroids.

Besides, the GnRH regulations occur through interference of central modulators, among which opiate peptides which should have an inhibitory effect in synergy with progesterone [18]. Alpha-adrenergic compounds accelerate the pulsatility induced by GnRH [19].

The hypothesis involving prostaglandins (PGs) is the most likely.

Thus, inhibitors of PGs-synthetases seem to be effective to treat certain symptoms of the premenstrual syndrome [2]. Fluctuations of PGF_2 or PGE_2 would favor vasodilatation and an increase in capillary permeability. PGE_2, PGF_2 and PGM are at rates notably lower in. Noradrenaline, serotonin, dopamine, stimulate the synthesis of PGs, which stimulation may involve a block of the dopaminergic receptors at the level of the central nervous system. PGs of E series contribute to the release of vasopressin, which involve a reduction in the urine ouptut and an hypermolarity of the urines, causing a premenstrual hydrosodic retention. PGE acts at the level of the androgenic control while PGF is under cholinergic control [20]. Whatever the favoring causes (hormones or PGs), clinically, we encounter the same effects : hydrosodic retention, hence weight gain, vasodilatation, increase in capillary permeability, generalized interstitial edema, of the breasts as well as peritoneal edema, or even cerebral edema.

Few groups have tried to use venotonic agents to treat premenstrual syndrome. However, all these clinical facts make it logical to think of substances which accelerate the venous return, act upon vessels and tissue congestion, are effective on lymphatics, without hormonal effects [21] and in addition having widely shown their harmlessness. This was done in a previous open study [22] using *Ruscus* in 3326 women [22]. We now report the results of a placebo-controlled, double-blind study with *Ruscus*.

Methods

The investigation was performed as a randomized double-blind study of *Ruscus*-extract against placebo. Twenty women were included in each group.

To be included, each patient should be between 18-50 years of age and suffer from premenstrual syndrome.

The exclusion criteria were : organic pathology, other gynaecological pathology, menopause, venotonic or hormonal co-treatments, other therapeutic study.

All patients received either placebo or *Ruscus*-extract as undifferentiated capsules, to be taken twice a day starting the first day after following monthly period (D0), ending 90 days after (D90). Additional visits were arranged at D30 and D60)

During each visit, the following criteria were investigated :

Efficacy :

Main criteria : breasts tension, pelvis heaviness, menstrual psychopathic disorder, ankle edema measurement.

Other criteria : telangectasia, menstrual flow regulation, menstrual pain, spotting, varicose veins.

The intensity of each criteria was marked : 0 (none); 1 (weak); 2 (medium); 3 (strong) except the edema that was measured in cm.

Tolerance :

It was asked if the patient had something to complain about and if adverse drug reaction had appeared during the study.

The population were compared in order to determine the group homogeneity. Statistical methods as Fisher or Chi-square test for qualitative item was used (number of pregnancies of impregnant, contraception, activity, previous history, previous therapy, etc.). Mean value (± S.D.) were calculated for quantitative items (age, weight, etc.). Treatment evaluation was performed at each consultation with Chi-square, and Fisher test for semi quantitative items and with Anova test for qualitative results (measurements).

Results

Population :

The whole population studied may be described as :

age : 27,5 years ± 0,28 (25-30)

weight : 58,3 kg ± 0,37 (55-65)

All patient had been pregnant, none of them was diabetic or having phlebitis. Their premenstrual syndrome trouble was going on for 67,5 months ± 0,68 (60–72).

Initial homogeneity :

At the beginning of the study, the two groups were found to be statistically similar in terms of characteristics of the population, selection or efficacy criteria.

Missing data

Few data were missing. This was equally divided between the two groups. All patients included reached the end of the study (D90).

Evaluation criteria

Breasts tension *(Figure 2)*, pelvis heaviness *(Figure 3)* and menstrual psychopathic disorder *(Figure 4)* show a significant difference between placebo and *Ruscus*-extract group (p < 0.05), *(Figure 7)*.

In terms of measurement of ankle edema *(Figure 1)*, the patients of *Ruscus*-extract group are more improved than those of the placebo group but this difference did not reach statistical significance.

Spotting and menstrual flow regulation results show borderline significant difference *(Figure 5 and 6)* whereas telangectasias and varicose veins were not different without improvement in either group.

The menstrual pain score in *Ruscus*-extract group decreased significantly (p < 0,005) *(Figure 7)*.

Tolerance

No adverse drug reactions were noted. Each treatment was well tolerated.

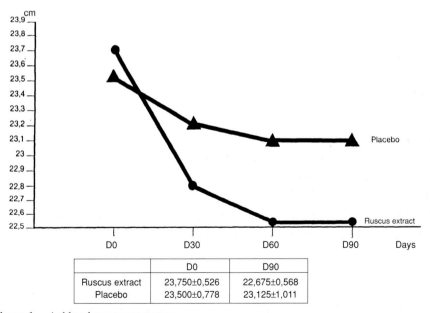

	D0	D90
Ruscus extract	23,750±0,526	22,675±0,568
Placebo	23,500±0,778	23,125±1,011

Figure 1. – Ankle edema measurement.

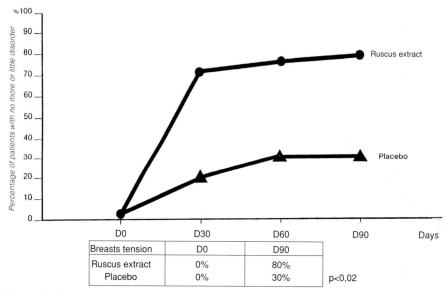

Breasts tension	D0	D90	
Ruscus extract	0%	80%	
Placebo	0%	30%	p<0,02

Figure 2. – Breasts tension.

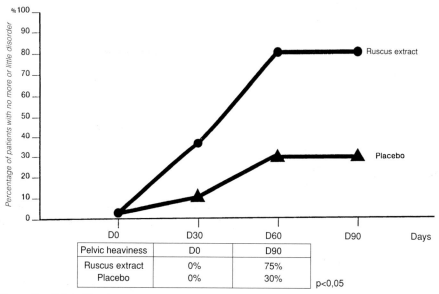

Pelvic heaviness	D0	D90	
Ruscus extract	0%	75%	
Placebo	0%	30%	p<0,05

Figure 3. – Pelvic Heaviness.

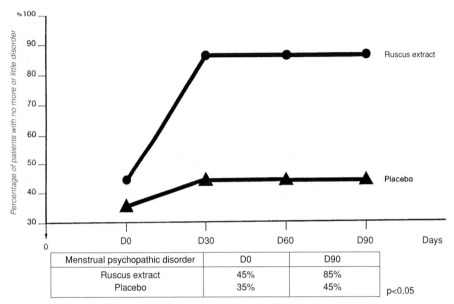

Menstrual psychopathic disorder	D0	D90
Ruscus extract	45%	85%
Placebo	35%	45%

p<0,05

Figure 4. – Menstrual psychopathic disorder.

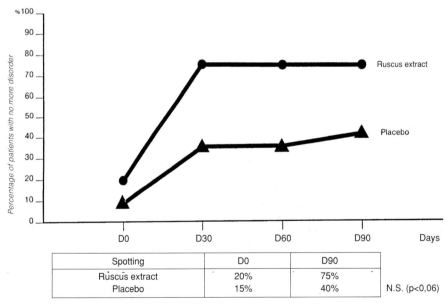

Spotting	D0	D90
Ruscus extract	20%	75%
Placebo	15%	40%

N.S. (p<0,06)

Figure 5. – Spotting.

49

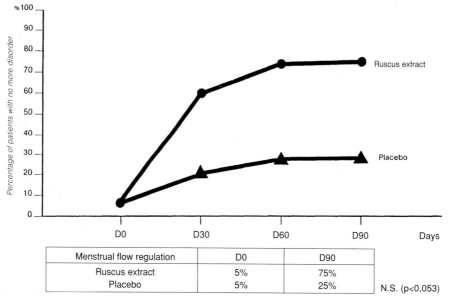

Figure 6. – Menstrual flow regulation.

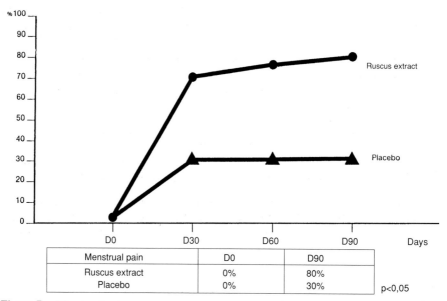

Figure 7. – Menstrual pain.

Discussion

The tol erance was very good, in confirmation of previous experience, which had enabled us to place it on an average and out of more than 10 000 cases, at 98.7 % [23]. Results of the active treatment are not surprising either. *Ruscus,* an alpha-adrenergic agonist [24], ameliorates the function of peripheral veins [16]. Its effects on the venous smooth muscle fibers (increase in tone), a decrease of the venous capacity and better cooptation of the valvules have been evidenced by Lauressergues [25]. Rudofsky [26] does not find the plethysmographic alterations, noted on subjects treated with placebo, in women treated with *Ruscus*-extract. Vanhoutte and Harker [27] have obtained with *Ruscus* much better venous contractions. The effects on the enzymes contained in the vein walls and necessary for the metabolism of adrenaline and noradrenaline have been established by Osswald [28]. At last, Marcelon *et al.* [29] have established that the best results of *Ruscus* were obtained at the end of the cycle.

However, some of our results require comments. The low efficacy of *Ruscus*-extract on varices and varicose veins is explained by a disappearance of the muscle fibers, a dystrophy of the elastic fibers and a fibrosis of the uterus at the anatomopathologic level. These findings are corroborated by Teixeira and Osswald [31], who showed in addition a drop of the extraneuronal uptake and enzymatic inactivation of catecholamines. Changes in noradrenaline metabolism have been confirmed by Branco [32]. Edema did not notably improved in comparison to the placebo group. This may be surprising since *Ruscus* does create a protection against edema, as evidenced by the different methods of Felix [33] and Potier [34]. However it is likely that the duration of the *Ruscus*-extract treatment in the present study was too short for this indication.

The improvement of psychic disorders was unexpected since *Ruscus* to our knowledge has no psychotropic or quieting effect. Hence, it must be that the drug acts by ameliorating the cerebral circulation — hence improving metabolism — which then results in the definite improvement noted.

As regards breast tension, the rapidity and the quality of the results seem to be clinical evidence for the improvement of the lymphatic component, which plays an essential role at the breast level, by *Ruscus*-extract. The tonic effect of *Ruscus* on the lymphatic system have been demonstrated by several investigators [35-37].

In addition, the cutaneous circulation of the breasts is important and *Ruscus* is more efficient on cutaneous than on deeper veins [38].

In conclusion, the results of *Ruscus*-extract in this study against placebo are superior to those we found in 1985, in an open study [22]. This could reflect both a better methodology and the fact that the open study had been carried out with a lesser dose of *Ruscus*-extract.

References

1. Franck RT. The hormonal causes of premenstrual tension. Archives of Neurology and Psychiatry 1931; 26 : 1053-1057.
2. Pariser SF, Stein SL, Shank ML *et al*. Premenstrual syndrome : causes, controversis and treatment. Am J Obst Gynecol 1985; 153 : 599-604.
3. Reid R, Yen SSC. Premenstrual syndrome. Am J Obst Gynecol 1981; 139 : 85-104.
4. Moos RH, Kopell BS, Melges FT *et al*. Fluctuations in symptoms and mood during the menstrual cycle. J Psychosom Res 1979; 13 : 37-44.
5. Dalton K. The premenstrual syndrome. William Heinsmann Medical books Ltd. London, 1984.
6. Lagrue G. Syndrome prémenstruel et syndrome d'œdème idiopathique orthostatique. Rev Sc Med 1975; 217.
7. Van Keep PA, Lehert Ph. Le syndrome prémenstruel. Contraception Fertilité Sexualité, 1980; 8, 10 : 775-779.
8. Netter A. Thérapeutique du syndrome prémenstruel. Sem Hôp, 12 Oct. 1960 ; 36, 47 : 2519-2520.
9. Magos AL, Brincot M, Studd JWW. Treatment of the premenstrual syndrome by subcutaneous oestradiol implants and cyclical oral norethisterone : placebo controlled study. British Medical Journal, 21 Juin 1986; 292; 1629-1633.
10. Muse KN. The premenstrual syndrome : effects of the medical ovariectomy. New England Journal of Medicine 1984; 311 : 1345-1349.
11. Hamarback S, Backstrom T. Induced anovulation as the treatment of premenstrual tension syndrome. A double blind cross-over study with Gn RH agonist versus placebo. Acta Obstet Gynecol Scand 1988; 67 : 159-166.
12. Lagrue G, Behar A, Morville R. Etude de la fonction ovarienne au cours des œdèmes idiopathiques orthostatiques. Presse Médicale, 10 Déc. 1983; 12, 45 : 2859-2862.
13. Steiner M, Haskett RF, Carroll BJ *et al*. Circadian hormone secretory profiles in women with severe premenstrual tension syndrome. British Journal Obstet Gynecol 1984 ; 91, 5 : 466-471.
14. Haskett RF. A psychoendocrine study of premenstrual tension syndrome. J of Affective disorders 1984; 6, 2 : 191-199.
15. Abraham GE. Nutritional factors in the etiology of the premenstrual syndrome. J Reprod Med 1983; 28 : 446-469.
16. Conclusion des 13e journées sur la fertilité et l'orthogénie. Paris, 9-11 Nov. 1989 (in press).

17. Vanhoutte PM. Control of venous function. International angiology 1984; 3, supp. 1 : 40-46

18. Wildt L, Martini L. 2e congrès européen de reproduction humaine et d'embryologie. Bruxelles 10-14 Juin 1986.

19. Lecomte P. Actualités concernant le cycle menstruel. Gynécologie 1988; 39 supp. 2 : 3-7.

20. Tourelle R. Antiprostaglandines et syndrome prémenstruel. La lettre du gynécologue 1989; suppl. 110 : 18-22.

21. Stenger J, Monteil-Seurin J. Recherche des propriétés œstrogènes du Cyclo 3. 1963, non publié.

22. Monteil-Seurin J. Aspects cliniques et intérêt du Clyclo 3 dans le traitement du syndrome prémenstruel. La vie médicale, Juillet/Août 1985.

23. Monteil-Seurin J. Value of *Ruscus* in gyneacological pathology, 25 years of use in private practice. Phlebology 1988; Vol. 3, suppl. 1 : 87-98.

24. Marcelon G., Vanhoutte PM. Mechanism of action of *Ruscus*-extract. International Angiology 1984; 3, suppl. 1 : 74-76.

25. Lauressergues H, Vilain P. Pharmacological activities of *Ruscus*-extracts on venous smooth muscle. International Angiology 1984; 3, suppl. 1 : 70-73.

26. Rudofsky G, Hirche H, Meyer P. Plethysmographic investigations of venous drug. Phlebology 1988; Vol. 3, suppl. 1 : 55-58.

27. Harker CT, Marcelon G, Vanhoutte PM. Temperature, œstrogen and contractions of the venous smooth muscle of the rabbit. Phlebology 1988; Vol. 3, suppl 1 : 77-82.

28. Osswald W. Enzymatic inactivation of catecholamines in the venous wall. International Angiology 1984; 3, suppl. 1 : 49-52.

29. Marcelon G, Vieu S, Pouget G, *et al.* Estrogenous impregnation and *Ruscus* action on the human vein *in vitro,* depending on preliminary results. Phlebology 1988 ; Vol. 3 ; suppl. 1 : 83-86.

30. Bouissou H, Julian M, Louge L, *et al.* Vein morphology. Phlebology 1988 ; Vol. 3, suppl. 1 : 1-12.

31. Teixeira AA, Osswald W. Effects of *Ruscus aculeatus* extract on the structural and functional alterations caused by sympathetic denervation of the saphenous vein. Phlebology 1988; Vol. 3, suppl. 1 : 27-32.

32. Branco D, Osswald W. The influence of *Ruscus*-extract on the uptake and metabolism of nor-adrenaline in the normal and varicose human saphenous vein. Phlebology 1988; Vol. 3, suppl. 1 : 33-40.

33. Felix W. Pharmacological models for the investigation of veinotropic drugs. International Angiology 1984; 3, suppl. 1 : 53-59.

34. Potier P. Relationship between chemical structure and pharmacological properties. International Angiology 1984; 3, suppl. 1 : 68-69.

35. Azevedo I, Teixeira A. Physio-pharmacology of the lymphatics. Phlebology 1988, Vol. 3, suppl 1 : 99-104.

36. Behar A. Pharmaco-clinical validation of models, protocols, results and applications. Phlebology 1988; Vol. 3, suppl. 1 : 113-120.

37. McHale NG. Neural control of lymphatic pumping. Phlebology 1988 ; Vol. 3, suppl. 1 : 105-108.

38. Flavahan NA, Vanhoutte PM. Thermo-sensitivity of cutaneous and deep veins. Phlebology 1988; Vol. 3, suppl. 1 : 41-46.

Return circulation and Norepinephrine : an update. Ed. P.M. Vanhoutte. John Libbey Eurotext, Paris © 1991, pp. 55-61.

5

First results with *Ruscus* extract* in the treatment of pregnancy related varicose veins

D. Berg

Ensinger Str. 1, 7900 Ulm, Germany

Thirty per cent of primigravidas and sixty per cent of multiparas suffer varicose changes in the veins during pregnancy. Varicosis is thus the most common form of vascular disease in pregnancy. Dilatation of the veins is associated with loss of function and edema, and frequently also with subjective complaints, such as feeling of heaviness or tension, or pain in the legs. The special haemodynamic situation during pregnancy produces a slowing of venous flow. Pregnancy varicosis therefore carries a risk that thrombosis and embolisms will occur.

The preventive measures used are kinesitherapy, applications of cold water, and compressive stockings. Although good results can be obtained with the drug treatment of varicosis, particularly in chronic venous insufficiency, there have as yet been relatively few studies of the use of drugs to control pregnancy varicosis. The reason for this may be that the range of diagnostic procedures and instrumental monitoring techniques that can be applied during pregnancy is very limited. With duplex B-scan sonography we now have a method that is completely safe for mother and child, and which makes it possible to detect venous dilatation in due time and to check the treatments used.

---

* Phlebodril® cream

Ruscus extract in combination with trimethylhesperidin chalcone or in combination with melilot extract has a venotonic action in clinical studies in volunteers [1-3] and in patients with chronic venous insufficiency [4]. At the same time, edema was reduced and the subjective complaints disappeared [5].

The increase in venous tone was demonstrated in these studies by venous occlusion plethysmography with occlusion pressures of 60-80 mm Hg. A direct determination of the action of *Ruscus* extract on vein diameter under orthostatic conditions was not possible until the introduction of duplex sonography.

Since the effect of *Ruscus* on venous diameter in orthostasis had not been studied the effect of single administrations of *Ruscus* extract was tested in healthy volunteers. As there was a significant reduction in vein diameter, in a follow-up study *Ruscus* extract was used to treat pregnancy varicosis and the associated subjective symptoms.

Patients and method

Volunteer study

The femoral vein diameter was determined in 18 volunteers aged 18-44 years. There were no externally discernible or known vein disorders. Eight volunteers were treated with a placebo and 10 with the active medication (cream).

The cross-section of the femoral vein was measured in the morning (8 a.m.) and 5 hours later in the afternoon, below the junction of the great saphenous vein, in standing position. Between the two measurements the volunteers were able to continue their normal daily activities.

Immediately after the morning measurement the lower legs and thighs of both legs were rubbed with 2-3 g cream. After 3 hours a further 2-3 g cream was applied to each leg, so that totally 4-6 g cream was applied to each leg, depending on the height of the volunteer.

100 g cream contain, as active constituents, 1.6 g *Ruscus* extract and 1.6 g melilot extract.

In the evaluation the means of vein diameters in the right and left legs were calculated. The effect of the treatment was checked on the basis of intraindividual differences in vein diameter between the value before and after treatment, using the Mann-Whitney U-test.

Pregnancy study

Nine pregnant women with clear pregnancy varicosis, aged 24-38 (median 29 years), have been enrolled in the study. They came to the surgery for the treatment of pain in the second trimester complaining of pains on only one side, generally the right.

As basic treatment all the patients received a compressive stocking and were told about the importance of further physical measures such as the application of cold water and kinesitherapy. In 3 patients the painful leg was also twice daily rubbed with *Ruscus* extract cream.

In the statistical evaluation Fisher's exact test was used to check whether, in the 3rd trimester of pregnancy the diameter of the femoral vein was greater in the painful leg than in the pain-free leg.

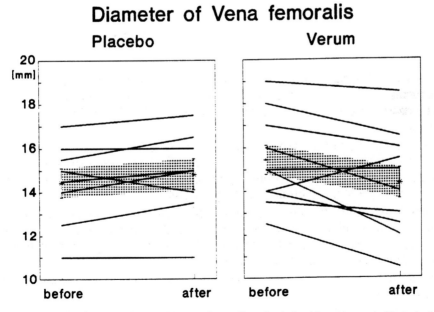

Figure 1. – Effect of cream application on femoralis veins in healthy volunteers (Dotted : the range of standard error).

Results

In healthy volunteers the mean diameter of the femoral vein was 15 mm. Male volunteers (diameter 16.1 mm) on average had a femoral vein 2 mm wider than the female volunteers (14.1 mm). In 8 of the 10 volunteers in the active medication group the diameter of the femoral vein decreased by between 0.5 and 3 mm (median 1.25 mm) as a result of the treatment, whereas in 7 volunteers in the placebo group the diameter remained constant or increased during the day (median of the increase 0.5 mm) *(Figure 1)*.

The difference between the two treatment groups is statistically significant (p = 0.0139).

In the pregnant women the diameter of the femoral vein in the painful leg was clearly greater than in the pain-free leg at the start of the treatment in the 2nd trimester. The difference was 1.6 mm in the patients who did not receive the cream treatment *(Figure 2)*. The slight difference in vein diameter between the painful and pain-free legs in the patients treated with cream in the 2nd trimester of pregnancy may be due to the fact that the measured value

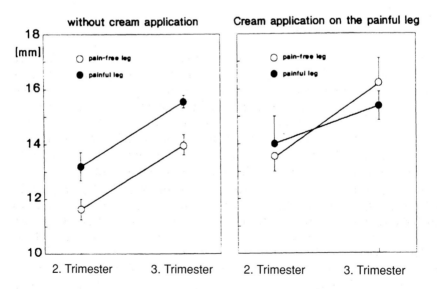

Figure 2. – Changes of diameter in femoralis veins in pregnant women (mean and standard error). The cream was only rubbed on the painful leg.

means were for the entire trimester, whereas treatment was started during the second trimester of pregnancy.

In the 3rd trimester of pregnancy it was seen that on treatment with cream the vein diameter increased far less than without the cream treatment, so that despite the fact that the treated side had originally shown more extensive varicosis in the 3rd trimester it showed a diameter almost 1 mm smaller than that of the untreated side. Despite the small number of patients, the differences in the increase in vein diameter are significant (Table I) ($p = 0.047$). At the same time the painful complaints were reduced.

Table I. – Differences in diameter of femoralis veins between painful and pain-free legs, 3rd trimester of pregnancy.

Treatment	Diameter painful leg > pain-free leg	Diameter painful leg ≤ pain-free leg
Without cream	5	1
Cream	0	3

$p = 0.0476$ Fisher's exact test, two-tailed.

Discussion

In healthy volunteers the diameter of the femoral veins decreased by 7 % within 2-2.5 h of application of the *Ruscus* extract, whereas under the placebo it increased by only 2-3 %. Thebault [6] and Rudofsky [7], using other study methods, also found a duration of action of at least 2.5 h. In their studies, however, the extensibility of the veins was reduced by 40 or 20 %. It must be borne in mind, though, that they were studying superficial veins with more pronounced musculature, whereas the measurements made here were of the deep vein system, which has a small proportion of smooth muscle.

A corresponding decrease in vein diameter was found by Ludwig [8] and by Ludwig and Glänzer [9] after oral administration of aescin. The route by which the active substances of the *Ruscus* extract reach the femoral vein was not established in this study. A systemic action would also be conceivable, as has been demonstrated by Thebault and Rudofsky after topical administration. It seems unlikely that *Ruscus* can penetrate the skin to a depth of 1-2 cm to reach the femoral vein. The result show, however, that the active substances of *Ruscus* extract penetrate the horny layer of the skin relatively quickly and to a sufficient degree, triggering and increase in venous tone. In animal experiments the hormone-induced reduced sensitivity of the α2-receptors was cancelled out by the administration of *Ruscus* extract. This led to a clear increase in venous tone [10]. A similar action mechanism can be assumed to operate in pregnant women, since in *in vitro* studies with human vein segments no change in tone was discernible after the administration of *Ruscus,* despite pretreatment with various estrogens [11]. This increase in tone may reduce the residual loss of function often observed after delivery.

An increase of 1-2 mm in vein diameter between the 2nd and 3rd trimesters is normal in pregnancy [12]. The small increase in vein diameter after treatment with *Ruscus* extract shows that the effect of increasing venous tension found after a single administration to healthy volunteers also occurs in long-term medication of patients with pregnancy varicosis.

The favourable effect on subjective symptoms reported by patients treated with cream was observed by Schröder in 30 pregnant women [9] and in a multicenter study [14] with 214 pregnant women. At the same time, a clear reduction in edema was found in these studies. The action of *Ruscus* extract observed as alleviation of subjective symptoms was confirmed in this study by measuring the reduction in vein diameter.

Animal studies have not produced any evidence of any embryotoxic action of *Ruscus* extract. Studies performed to date in pregnant women have likewise not yielded any such evidence. The combination of *Ruscus* extract with melilot extract or with trimethylhesperidin chalcone is therefore suitable for the support of basic therapy in patients with pregnancy varicosis or for the treatment of chronic venous insufficiency in pregnant women.

References

1. Rudofsky G, Nobbe F. Zur Wirkung eines Kombinationspräparates auf die Venenkapazität. Fortschr Med 1982; 100 (25) : 1217-1220.
2. Rudofsky G, Hirche H. Plethysmographische Untersuchungen eines Venentherapeutikums bei wärmebedingten hämodynamischen Veränderungen. Med Welt 1985; 36 : 145-149.
3. Rudofsky G. Venentonisierung und Kapillarabdichtung. Fortschr Med 1989 ; 107 (19) : 430-434.
4. Rudofsky G. Plethysmographic studies of venous capacity and venous outflow and venotropic therapy. Inter Angio 1984; 3, Suppl. 1 : 95-98.
5. Rudofsky G, Diehm C, Gruß J, *et al.* Wirksamkeit einer Kombination venoaktiver Substanzen bei Patienten mit chronisch-venöser Insuffizienz im Stadium I. *In* Denk H, RJAM van Dongen (eds), *Therapie der Venenerkran-kungen* 1989; 73-92, TM-Verlag, Hameln.
6. Thebault JJ. Untersuchungen zur Wirkung eines Phlebotonikums. Fortschr Med 1983 ; 25 : 101 Jg, 1206-1212.
7. Rudofsky G. Ruscus-Extrakt - Transkutane Venentonisierung und Kapillarabdichtung bei gesunden Probanden. MMW 1989; 18 : 131 Jg, 362-365.

8. Ludwig M. Bestimmung des Venenquerschnitts mit Hilfe des Zweidimensionalen Ultra-schalle. Phlebol. u. Proktol. 16, 229-30 (1987).

9. Ludwig M., Glänzer K. Die Bestimmung der Querschnittsfläche und der Blutströmungs-geschwindigkeit in der Vena femoralis mit Hife der Duplexsonographie - Eine Möglich-keit zur Wirkung von Venentherapeutika. VASA, Suppl. 20, 8, 328 (1987).

10. Harker C.T., Marcelon G., Vanhoutte P.M. Temperature, oestrogens and contractions of venous smooth muscle o the rabbit. Phlebology (1988) 3, Suppl. 1, 77-82.

11. Marcelon G., Vieu S., Pouget G., Tisné-Versailles J. Oestrogenous impregnation and *Ruscus* action on the human vein *in vitro,* depending on preliminary results.

12. Sohn Ch., Rudofsky G. Veränderungen am Beinvenensystem in der Schwangerschaft. Fortschr. Med. 106 (17), 351-354 (1988).

13. Schröder F.A. Phlebodril-Creme bei schwangerschaftsvarikosis. Extracta gynaecologica 9 (2), 151-172 (1985).

14. Leutenegger S., Martinaggi P. Cyclo 3 fort et grossesse. Gazette Médicale 95 (33) (1988).

Return circulation and Norepinephrine : an update. Ed. P.M. Vanhoutte. John Libbey Eurotext, Paris © 1991, pp. 63-71.

6

Therapeutic test of *Ruscus* extract* in pregnant women : evaluation of the fetal tolerance applying the pulse Doppler's method of the cord

J.H. Baudet, D. Collet, Y. Aubard, P. Renaudie

Gynecologic of obstetric Department, University Hospital Dupuytren, 87042 Limoges cedex.

Introduction

The frequent occurence of disturbances ascribed to a venous drainage insufficiency at the level of the lower limbs in pregnant women, is such that it seemed useful to study the means to alleviate the symptoms, in particular the sensation of "heavy legs". Among the useful therapeutic methods we have chosen to carry out the therapeutic test of *Ruscus* extract.

Purpose of the test

The purpose of this therapeutic test is to evaluate the efficacy of *Ruscus* extract on venous symptoms occurring frequently during the two last quarters week of pregnancy. However, the most important part of the work consisted

---

* Cyclo 3 Fort®

in assessing the tolerance of this therapy not only by the mother but also by the foetus : therefore we chose the pulse Doppler's method of the cord which enables short or long range assessment of the exchanges between mother and infant.

Methodology

We chose, among the pregnant women consulting in our department soon at the beginning of their pregnancy, 20 women answering to following criteria:

Inclusion criteria

Women aged from 18 to 40 years.

Alleging symptoms which can be attributed to a venolymphatic insufficiency in the lower limbs : sensation of heavy legs, impression of swelling exaggerated by fatigue, dysesthesia or pains such as cramps and tension, minor disturbances of the venous pathology such as varicose veins or small venous dilatation without valvular insufficiency.

All these women were willing to participate to the study. They were informed about the methods employed and the objective aimed at.

Exclusion criteria

Ages under 18 or above 40 years.

Absence of the basic symptom of "heavy legs sensation".

Presence of signs giving evidence of a major venous pathology such as important varices with valvular insufficiency, clear trophic disturbances of varicose ulcer type or purpuric pigmented dermatis of Favre and Chaix, important and permanent edema of the lower limbs.

Severe pathology associated to pregnancy such as congestive heart failure or renal failure, acrocyanosis, Raynaud's syndrome, presence of sural phlebitis or of previous sural phlebitis.

Previous surgical intervention on varices dating less than one year back.

Treatment with other phlebotonics.

Previous intolerancy to *Ruscus* extract or acquired conviction of the physician and/or the patient about the inefficacy of such therapeutics.

For psychological reasons, we gave up proposing the therapeutic test to pregnant women with antecedents of multiple abortions or births of malformated infants, as well as to patients in whom we noticed a reticence, however light it might be, for such a test.

The study was constructed as an open trial carried out between May 1988 and May 1989.

Evaluation criteria

As always during a pregnancy, our attention was concentrated on the two beings interested in this symbiotic development : mother and infant.

The criteria with the mother concerned signs of venolymphatic insufficiency at the level of the lower limbs.

Following symptoms were taken into account : functional signs (sensation of heavy legs, pains, dysesthesia, cramp sensation, swelling sensation, and physical signs (smaller varices or varicose veins, smaller trophic disturbances, edema).

Evaluation of the therapeutic effect of *Ruscus* extract on all these symptoms was established as a whole by investigation of the pregnant women at the end of the treatment, using a three grade scale : average efficacy, good efficacy, excellent efficacy.

Maternal tolerance was appraised as a whole, using the same scale : average, good, excellent.

The study of the fetal tolerance evaluation which remains the most important part of the study was performed in detail.

Besides the clinical criteria, which belong to the usual surveillance of a pregnancy (gain in weight of the mother, arterial pressure, proteinuria, glycosuria, height of the fundus uteri, fetal active movements, presence or absence of contractions), we have collected the ultrasonographic criteria with the fetal biometry (ultrasonographies at 7-8 weeks, 12 weeks, 17-18 weeks, 22 or 24 weeks, 32 or 34 weeks, 36 or 37 weeks and 40 or 41 weeks). All these information enabled us to estimate the regular and harmonious growth of the foetus.

When expressing our results, we noted the absence of clinical or ultrasonographic pathological facts concerning the evolution of each of the pregnancies.

However, we wanted to go further into the foetus exploration in order to demonstrate the lack of unwanted effects of *Ruscus* extract. Therefore, we used the pulse Doppler's method on the umbilical cord.

We used an ultrasonographic set provided with a Doppler's sound and a screen on which we displayed the spectral analysis. The spectral analysis of the obtained signal permits independent index calculation of the Doppler's beam angle of bank on the axis of the vessel size. We can thus distinguish two components per heart cycle, a diastolic one (D) of minimal velocity, directly influenced by the peripheral resistance, and a systolic one (S) of maximal velocity reflecting the heart ejection power.

Among the different proposed indexes we chose Pourcelot's index : (S-D)/S. It is proportional to the resistance to flow exerted by the vascular bed located downstream of the studied vessel.

During a normal pregnancy, we observe a progressive rise of the diastolic flows at the level of the umbilical cord, hence a decrease of Pourcelot's index. Any increase of Pourcelot's index means an increase in the resistance to the blood flow at the level of the placenta, that is, all things considered, a decrease of the possibilities of oxygen exchanges and nutrition from mother to infant.

Pourcelot's index increase is a very good means to detect chronical fetal pain even before its clinical manifestations (growth delay *in utero*). It is known that when the diastolic flows become negative (Pourcelot's index = 1), the fetal prognosis is bad and the danger of fetal death *in utero* is high. On the other hand, in essential uterine hypotrophia, where Doppler's test of the umbilical cord is normal, we know that a light weight of the newborn infant does not involve serious neonatal consequences.

Taking into account the normal evolution of Pourcelot's index during a normal pregnancy, we decided to measure it a first time, before any treatment with *Ruscus* extract, after 21 to 24 weeks of gravidic amenorrhea (WGA) and a second time, after 6 weeks at least and 13 weeks at most of continuous treatment with *Ruscus* extract on the basis of two capsules per day.

Ultimately we collected a certain amount of information concerning the delivery and the infant's state at birth :

— Length of the pregnancy in weeks of amenorrhea

— Weight of the newborn infant

— Apgar's index

— Anatomopathological investigation of the placenta.

Results

Studied population

We included in this study 20 pregnant women having a normal pregnancy by the time the investigation was started.

Ages ranged from 19 to 38 (*Figure 1*) : fifteen of our patients were located within an age bracket between 24 and 32 years. Only one was under 20 years. The four oldest ones were aged between 34 and 38 years.

Parity was as follows : 9 primiparae, 5 secundiparae and 6 third parae.

This test did not include big multiparae.

Antecedents and exclusion criteria led us to eliminate women having an associated pathology which might influence the normal progress of pregnancy. However, we noted a particular observation : antecedent of preeclampsia syndrome during the former pregnancy, corresponding to a pure gravidic hypertension which did not recur during the studied pregnancy.

The last pregnancy check-up, before starting up the test, was in all cases normal from a clinical point of view as well as from the ultrasonographic one.

The treatment follow-up has always been satisfactory, except in one case where, because of a few *Ruscus* extract omissions, it was qualified as "average".

In eight cases, other treatments were prescribed in addition to *Ruscus* extract.

1st case : magnesium, metoclopramide, salbutamol, dehydro-progesterone

2nd case : metoclopramide

3rd case : magnesium, ferrous sulphate

4th case : indomethacine

5th case : dipyridamol, aspirin

6th, 7th and 8th cases : magnesium

Yet such therapies do not allert the principle of single therapy prescribed for venolymphatic disturbances.

The symptoms which led to the prescribtion of *Ruscus* extract were classed in 5 items : sensation of heavy legs, 19 cases, pain in the lower limbs, 17 cases, swelling of the lower limbs exaggerated by fatigue, 4 cases, dysesthesia, tension sensation, cramp type pain, 13 cases, venous pathology (varicose veins, edema, venous dilatation without valvular insufficiency), 17 cases.

It thus emerges from our study that, in a majority of cases, patients treated with *Ruscus* extract complain from a sensation of heavy legs with pain in the lower limbs, dysesthesia appearing on a background on minor venous pathology, apart from cases of real varices with valvular insufficiency and serious trophic disturbances.

Evaluation of the therapeutic results in mother

The efficacy of the therapy with *Ruscus* extract was evaluated as follows :
very good efficacy, 9 cases; good efficacy, 11 cases.
"Very good efficacy" means that, by each of the alleged symptoms, the patient felt a highly satisfactory improvement. "Good efficacy" means that the patients are satisfied with the treatment, although all the symptoms of which they complained had not disappeared (e.g. small trophic disturbances and varicose veins would persist while functional disorders were improved).

Evaluation of the maternal tolerance

In 12 cases, maternal tolerance to the therapy has been assessed as " very good ". In 8 cases, it has been considered as " good " because the patients were complaining about a sensation of post-prandial digestive heaviness, ascribed to (although it is not possible to prove it) the therapy with *Ruscus* extract. In not a single case, we observed a drop out of therapy because of serious digestive disturbances or allergic accident.

It is thus possible to state that the tolerance of *Ruscus* extract by pregnant women, at the second quarter of the pregnancy, is satisfactory.

Evaluation of the foetal tolerance

The clinical criteria join together all surveillance details of a pregnancy. We have added the ultrasonographic criteria. Before the test began, every pregnant woman to whom we proposed it, had normal clinical and ultrasonographic investigations testifying to a regular and harmonious growth of the foetus, while the surveillance test carried out further on, every five weeks, confirmed this favorable development.

The birth fetal criteria were as follows : in 19 cases, the delivery took place normally, and in 1 case, a caesarean section was performed because of postmaturity. (This low rate of caesarean sections in the present study can be explained by the fact that the selected patients were free from all gravidic or pregnancy associated pathologies.)

The weight of the newborn infants was as follows : in one case, we had a premature childbirth after 36 weeks of gravidic amenorrhea, weight of the infant : 1950 grams. Yet, the infant's state was satisfactory as shown by Apgar's index (9 at the first minute, 10 at 5 and 10 minutes). In all other cases, delivery occurred at the end of a normal gestation period (except in the case of postmaturity). The weights at birth range from 2690 grams to 3650 grams : 5 infants weighed from 2690 to 2980 grams, 6 infants weighed from 3000 to 3200 grams, 8 infants weighed from 3200 to 3650 grams.

The Apgar's indexes measured at birth at 1 mn, 5 mn and 10 mn were normal (index equal or superior to 8 at 1 mn ; index equal or superior to 9 at 5 mn ; index equal to 10 at 10 mn). It is considered that Apgar's index is pathologic and testifies to fetal pain if it is inferior to 7.

In the end we used Doppler's velocimetry method of the umbilical artery to investigate whether there might be a change in the maternofetal transmission, as a consequence of the intake of *Ruscus* extract during pregnancy.

The *Table I* shows, for each case, the dates of the first and second tests in weeks of gravidic amenorrhea together with the values of Pourcelot's index at each of these dates.

In one case we made 3 Doppler's tests and in another case, 4 Doppler's tests were performed. The results are the following ones :

23 S.A.G. : 0,7. 29 S.A.G. : 0,68. 33 S.A.G. : 0,61.

21 S.A.G. : 0,71. 26 S.A.G. : 0,65. 31 S.A.G. : 0,68. 36 S.A.G. : 0,58.

However, the multiplication of these Doppler's velocimetric tests did not

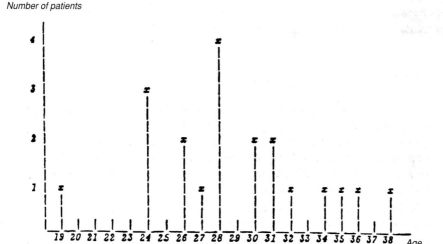

Figure 1. – Age range.

Table I. – Date of first and second tests of Doppler's velocitometry method and Pourcelot's index.

1st Doppler's test		2nd Doppler's test	
S.A.G.	I.P.	S.A.G.	I.P.
23	0,7	32	0,5
23	0,69	35	0,6
21	0,75	31	0,5
24	0,62	33	0,55
21	0,65	32	0,5
23	0,72	33	0,66
21	0,59	33	0,5
22	0,68	31	0,54
23	0,7	29	0,68
24	0,65	32	0,69
21	0,71	31	0,68
23	0,66	31	0,5
22	0,7	32	0,66
22	0,71	32	0,66
22	0,70	32	0,45
22	0,71	35	0,5
24	0,64	35	0,5
23	0,57	35	0,54
24	0,8	35	0,55
24	0,65	34	0,58

change the general profile of the study. These figures clearly show that Pourcelot's index was normal, in all cases, before the beginning of the treatment, what corresponds to the inclusion criteria of the patients. It appears, particularly, that after 9 to 10 weeks of treatment with *Ruscus* extract, Pourcelot's index remained normal in all cases.

Conclusion

This therapeutic trial, on 20 cases taking two capsules per day of *Ruscus* extract, after 21 to 24 weeks of gravidic amenorrhea, for simple veinolymphatic disturbances of the lower limbs, shows :

— An improvement of the pregnant women's relief, assessed according to subjective criteria.

— An absolute harmlessness for the infant, assessed with the usual clinical and ultrasonographic criteria of pregnancy surveillance, with Doppler's velocimetry at the level of the umbilical artery and with the state of the infant and the anatomopathologic aspect of the placenta after birth.

Return circulation and Norepinephrine : an update. Ed. P.M. Vanhoutte. John Libbey Eurotext, Paris © 1991, pp. 73-88.

7

Mechanism of noradrenaline action in lymphatic vessels

N.G. McHale

School of Biomedical Science (Physiology), The Queen's University of Belfast, 97 Lisburn Road, Belfast BT9 7BL, United Kingdom.

Introduction

Lymphatic vessels have been shown to be spontaneously contractile in almost all mammals that have been studied including man, horse, sheep, mouse, rat, guinea-pig, rabbit, squirrel, bat and dog [1-4]. In a few studies where intrinsic contractions were not observed anaesthesia or tissue trauma may have obscured the normal contractile activity of the lymphatics [1, 2]. It is likely, therefore, that intrinsic contractility of lymph ducts is a universal feature of the mammalian lymphatic system. Smith [5] argued persuasively that intrinsic lymphatic contractility was an important means by which lymph was propelled. He reasoned that even if lymph were propelled from the extremities by passive movement it would remain pooled in the proximal freely distensible lymphatics of the leg and thigh in the absence of an intrinsic propulsive mechanism. Experiments done in this laboratory [6, 7] and in others [8, 9] confirm the existence of such a pump which can be controlled in a variety of different ways. It will respond to an acute increase in fluid load by increasing the frequency and force of lymphatic contraction [6, 7] while Uhley and his colleagues [10] have shown that when they induced chronic heart failure in dogs the lymphatic system responded to the sustained increase in fluid load both by hypertrophy of individual vessels and by a proliferation in the number of vessels. This made it possible to increase lymph flow 25 times above normal. Lymphatic motility can also be modified by a variety of blood and lymph borne substances such as bradykinin, serotinin [11, 12] inflammatory mediators [12] and by catecholamines [13, 14]. Lymphatic vessels are innervated by noradrenergic nerves [15] stimulation of which increases the frequency of their spontaneous contractions and thus their pumping output [16, 17]. This review seeks to examine the way in which noradrenaline is released from these nerves and the mechanism of its action on lymphatic smooth muscle.

Noradrenaline release

This was investigated [18] by incubating the vessels with tritiated noradrenaline and monitoring its efflux in response to stimulation of the intramural nerves using the technique described by Su and Bevan [19]. *Figure 1* shows the effect when the vessels were stimulated at frequencies of 0.25, 1, 4 and 8 Hz (0.3 msec pulses, 40 V nominal, 1 min train). Spontaneous contraction rate and force were increased in proportion to stimulus frequency. The middle panel shows corresponding ^3H flux in d.p.m. Stimulation at 0.25, 1, 4 and 8 Hz caused a progressively larger increase in ^3H overflow with increasing stimulus frequency. The bottom panel summarizes the average of six such experiments where ^3H efflux is plotted as a percentage of the total ^3H tissue content at the time of stimulation. When these results were calculated on an output per pulse basis transmitter release increased in the range 0.25 to 4Hz but reached a maximum between 4 and 16Hz. ^3H efflux was potentiated by cocaine, by phentolamine (*Figure 2*) and by the α_2 antagonist yohimbine and inhibited by noradrenaline and the α_2 agonist xylazine but it was little affected by either the α_1 agonist phenylephrine or the α_2 antagonist prazosin (*Figure 3*) suggesting the presence of presynaptic α_2 receptors capable of regulating noradrenaline release. That a facilitatory presynaptic regulatory mechanism also exists is indicated by the experiment [20] shown in *Figure 4*. The upper record of this figure shows the efflux of ^3H (in d.p.m.) from a single lymphatic vessel. Under control conditions field stimulation (S1) evoked a distinct rise in ^3H efflux as before. At the time indicated, isoprenaline $10^{-6}M$ was introduced and remained for the rest of the experiment. While isoprenaline did not itself affect basal ^3H efflux, that released by the second period of field stimulation (S2) was clearly potentiated. The lower panel of this figure summarizes the results of five such experiments. Efflux is expres-

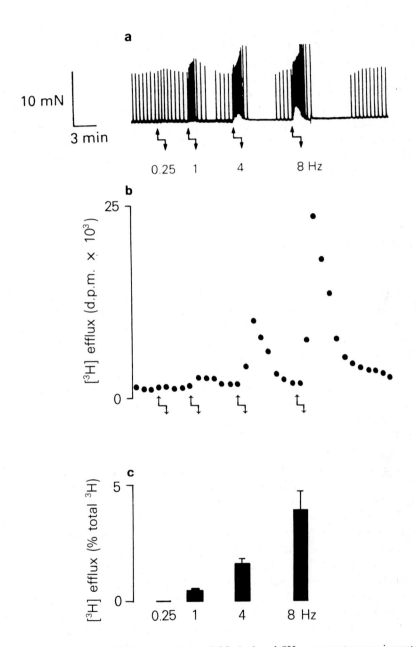

Figure 1. – The effect of field stimulation at 0.25, 1, 4 and 8Hz on spontaneous isometric contractions (top), the corresponding ^{3}H efflux in d.p.m. and the mean ^{3}H efflux for six experiments of this type plotted as a percentage of total tissue ^{3}H (from reference 18, with permission).

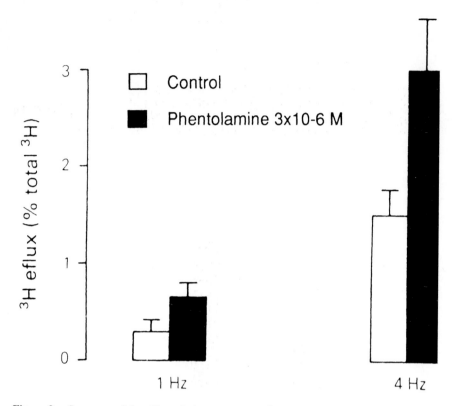

Figure 2. – Summary of the effect of phentolamine on ^{3}H (efflux expressed as a percentage of the total tissue content) in response to field stimulation at 1 and 4 Hz. Vertical lines represent SEM n=7 (from reference 18, with permission).

sed as a percentage of the total ^{3}H in the tissue at the time of stimulation. Isoprenaline significantly (p<0.05, paired t-test) increased field stimulated release of ^{3}H (S2/S1 = 1.8).

Mechanism of action

The results of the above study [18] also suggest that the predominant postsynaptic receptor type is α_2. Note, for example, in the top panel of *Figure 3*

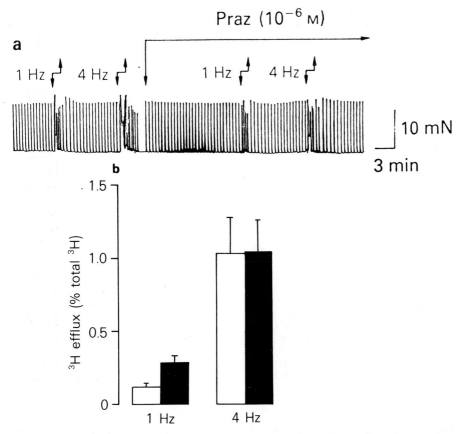

Figure 3. – The effect of Prazosin on (a) spontaneous contraction and (b) ^{3}H efflux as a percentage of the total tissue content. The open columns represent the effects of field stimulation before and the solid columns during prazosin treatment. Vertical lines represent SEM n=4 (from reference 18, with permission).

that prazosin had very little effect on the excitatory effect of field stimulation in contrast to the action of non selective a blockers [15] or the α_2 blockers yohimbine and rauwolscine [18] where the excitatory effect was converted to β inhibitory one. In an attempt to elucidate the mechanism of these effects Allen *et al.* [21, 22] and McHale *et al.* [23] used the double sucrose gap technique to study the changes at membrane level in response to α and β stimulation of lymphatic smooth muscle. Noradrenaline either alone or in the presence of the β blocker propranolol depolarized the membrane and increased the frequency of firing of action potentials. *Figure 5* shows a simultaneous electrical (upper record) and mechanical (lower record) recording from a bovine mesenteric lymphatic strip. Under control conditions there is a

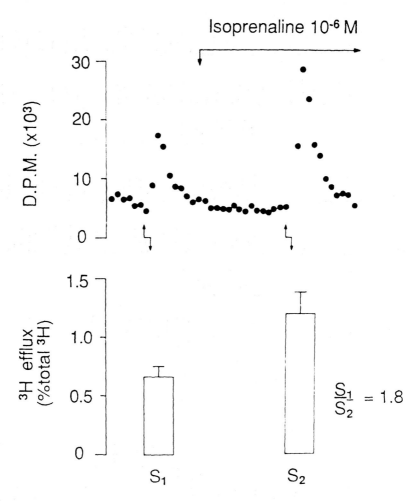

Figure 4. – The upper record shows the effect of isoprenaline on ^{3}H efflux in one experiment. Six such experiments are summarized as percentage total tissue ^{3}H in the lower record (from reference 20, with permission).

one to one correspondence between action potential firing and contraction. The depolarizatin caused by noradrenaline increased the frequency of spontaneous contractions in tandem with the increase in action potential firing except at the higher dose where some fusion of contractions occurred. When constant current pulses were applied across the stimulating gap in order to estimate changes in membrane resistance during noradrenaline perfusion, the size of the resulting hyperpolarizing electrotonic potential was increased as

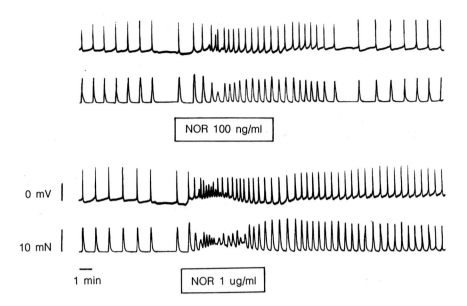

Figure 5. – The effect of noradrenaline on electrical (upper record) and (mechanical) activity recorded by the sucrose gap technique (from reference 21, with permission).

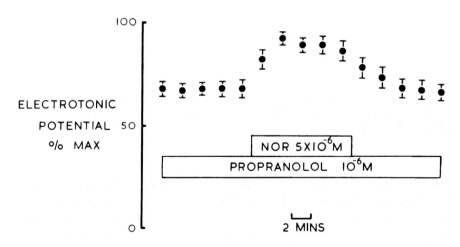

Figure 6. – Summary of the effect of noradrenaline on the size of the hyperpolarizing electrotonic potential in 15 lymphatics. Each point represents the mean ± SEM plotted as a percentage of maximum for each vessel (from reference 22, with permission).

shown in *Figure 6*. This decrease in membrane conductance in conjunction with a depolarization can best be explained by the shutting off of an outward current which is likely to be carried by K$^+$ ions. Stimulation of β receptors with isoprenaline had the opposite effect to that of the noradrenaline-propranolol combination. Frequency of spontaneous action potential firing was decreased *(Figure 7)* and this was accompanied by a hyperpolarization which was more marked at the higher dose, when action potential firing was completely inhibited. The effect of constant current pulses of alternating polarity is shown in *Figure 8*. Depolarizing pulses evoked action potentials in control conditions but during the application of isoprenaline 10^{-7}M these were abolished and this was accompanied by a decrease in the hyperpolarizing electronic potential. Five such experiments are summarized in *Figure 9* both before and after the addition of 10 mM tetraethylammonium. The decrease in membrane resistance produced by isoprenaline was significantly reduced by TEA suggesting that we are looking at an increase in an outward potassium current. The nature of the K$^+$ channels that might be involved in such a mechanism has not elucidated but recent work by Sadoshima *et al.* [24] has demonstrated a Ca^{2+} activated K$^+$ channel in rat aortic smooth muscle which is activated by cyclic AMP. McHale *et al.* [25] have described a channel with similar voltage and calcium dependent activation in canine lymphatic

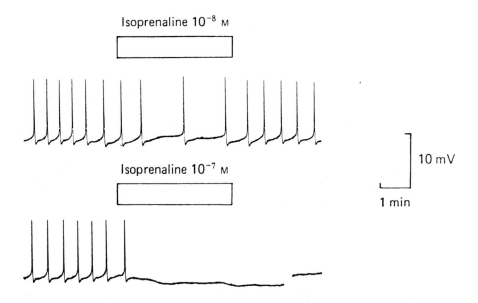

Figure 7. – The effects of two doses of isoprenaline on spontaneous electrical activity (from reference 23, with permission).

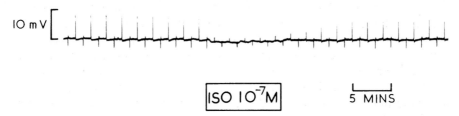

Figure 8. – The effects of isoprenaline on action potentials evoked by depolarizing pulses and on the size of the hyperpolarizing electrotonic potential (from reference 23, with permission).

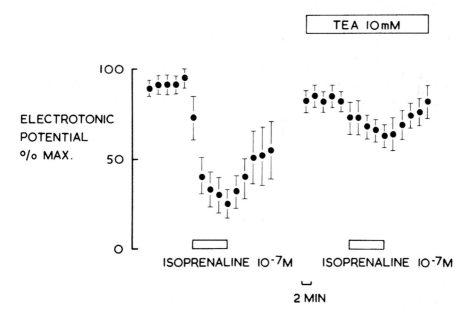

Figure 9. – A summary of the effect of isoprenaline on the size of the hyperpolarizing electrotonic potential in five experiments under control conditions (left hand panel) and in the presence of TEA (right hand panel). Each point is expressed as a percentage of the maximum value for each lymphatic (from reference 23, with permission).

smooth muscle. *Figure 10* shows a record of an experiment on an inside out patch taken from a freshly dispersed canine thoracic duct cell. In symmetrical 140 mM K^+ solutions at a holding potential of 40 mV there was little channel activity when the bath solution contained 10^{-7} M Ca^{2+} solution.

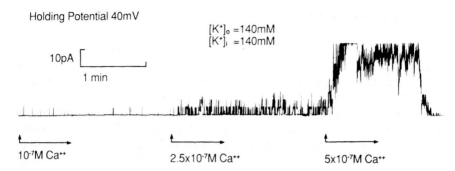

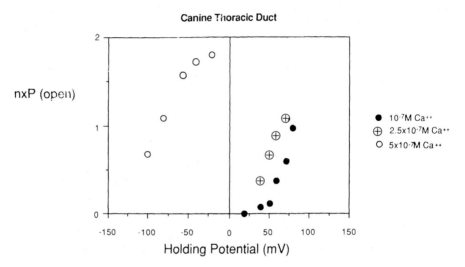

Figure 10. – Single channel recordings in an " inside out " patch of a lymphatic smooth muscle cell from the canine thoracic duct. The effect of changing the Ca^{2+} concentration at the inside of the membrane.

Figure 11. – Activation curves from an experiment such as that shown in fig 10 at three different calcium concentrations.

Activity increased markedly when the Ca^{2+} content of the bath solution was increased to 2,5 x 10^{-7} M with three channels discernible. Further increasing the calcium to 5 x 10^{-7} M resulted in an enormous increase in activity. *Figure 11* shows the activation curves for the three Ca^{2+} concentrations showing that at normal resting potential (about –60 mV) and at normal resting $[Ca^{2+}]_i$ these channels would rarely be in the open state.

Receptor desensitization

When the sympathetic chain is stimulated in the sheep there is an increase in popliteal efferent lymph flow [16]. If stimulation is sustained for more than ten or fifteen minutes the lymph flow response declines rapidly even though blood vessel constriction is maintained. Because of the complexities of whole animal experiments, it is not clear whether this is a fundamental difference in the nature of lymphatic and blood vascular innervation or an indirect effect due, for example, to decreased entry of fluid into the terminal

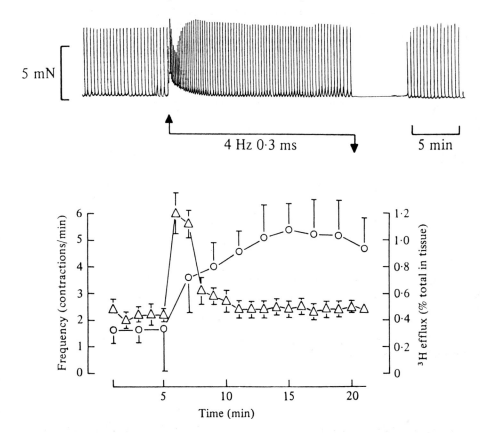

Figure 12. – The upper panel shows the effect of a 20 min period of field stimulation (period between the arrows). The lower panel shows a summary of the effect of field stimulation on contraction frequency (open triangles) and on 3H efflux (open circles). The open triangles represent mean frequency (n=10) of contraction averaged over the preceding minute while the open circles represent mean 3H efflux expressed as a percentage of the total tissue content in seven experiments (right axis) (from reference 26, with permission).

lymphatics secondary to depressed capillary filtration. When bovine ducts are stimulated *in vitro* a similar transient response to stimulation of the intramural nerves is seen [26]. The upper panel in *Figure 12* shows a record from such a preparation. In the control period the vessel was contracting with fairly consistent force and at a frequency of 2.8 contractions per minute. At the point shown by the first arrow field stimulation at 4Hz was applied and lymphatic contraction frequency immediately increased almost threefold during the first minute. Thereafter, however, frequency rapidly declined so that within ten minutes it was at 3.1/min almost back to control level. When the stimulation was switched off, at the point shown by the second arrow, spontaneous activity ceased for more than five minutes after which it returned at approximately control frequency. Ten such experiments are shown summarized in the lower panel of *Figure 12*. The open triangles represent the mean frequency of contraction averaged over the preceding minute. In the control period (first five points) mean frequency was about 2.2 contractions/min. In response to field stimulation this rose to nearly 6/min and then rapidly declined until, within six minutes of the beginning of stimulation, contraction frequency was no longer significantly different from control. It could be argued that the decline in lymphatic contraction frequency noted above was due to rapid exhaustion of noradrenaline stores in the nerve terminals of these isolated vessels. To find out if this were so, vessels which had been pre-incubated with ^{3}H noradrenaline were subjected to sustained stimulation. Superimposed on the frequency results in the lower panel of *Figure 12* is a summary of seven such experiments. The circles represent mean ^{3}H efflux expressed as a percentage of the total tissue content (right axis). In contrast to the effect on frequency ^{3}H efflux rose gradually during the first ten minutes and was maintained at a value significantly higher than control during the remainder of the stimulation period.

If, as these results suggest, the adaptation to field stimulation is a post-synaptic phenomenon one might expect that it could be mimicked by application of exogenous noradrenaline. This expectation was fulfilled as the experiment illustrated in *Figure 13* demonstrates. At the point shown by the first arrow the Krebs solution was replaced by one containing 10^{-6}M noradrenaline. Contraction frequency increased from a control value of about 2/min to a peak of 6/min but then rapidly returned to control. If the fade in contraction frequency during prolonged application of noradrenaline were due to desensitization of adrenoceptors and if these same receptors respond to endogenously released transmitter then it should be possible to block the effects of field stimulation by prior treatment with noradrenaline. This proved to be the case since after desensitization with noradrenaline, field stimulation at a frequency of 4 Hz was almost totally blocked. The extract of *Ruscus aculeatus* behaved differently from noradrenaline for, although it had a similar excita-

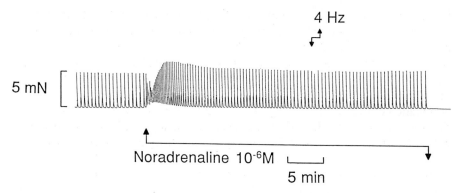

Figure 13. – The response to exogenous noradrenaline faded almost as rapidly as that to field stimulation. When the vessel was stimulated at 4 Hz (between the arrows) the response was almost totally abolished (from reference 26, with permission).

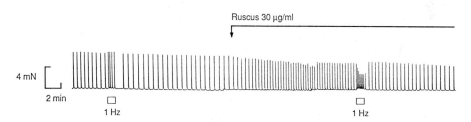

Figure 14. – The effect of field stimulation at 1 Hz before and after the addition of *Ruscus* extract. In contrast to the response in noradrenaline the effect of field stimulation was potentiated rather than blocked.

tory effect, this was sustained for the duration of drug perfusion. Furthermore instead of desensitizing the vessel to nerve stimulation it appeared rather to potentiate it. *Figure 14* shows an experiment where a bovine mesenteric lymphatic was stimulated at 1 Hz under control conditions. This resulted in a two fold increase in contraction frequency. On addition of *Ruscus* extract 30 μg/ml contraction frequency increased by about 50 % and this frequency was maintained until the 1 Hz stimulus was repeated. The second period of field stimulation produced a response which was greater than that of the control period. *Figure 15* shows a summary of six noradrenaline experiments (lower panel) and eight *Ruscus* experiments. Whereas the effect of sustained noradrenaline infusion was to block the response to field stimula-

85

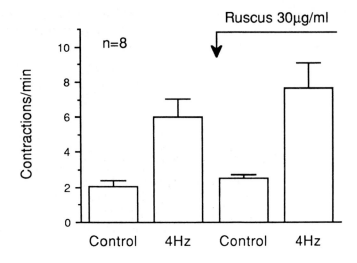

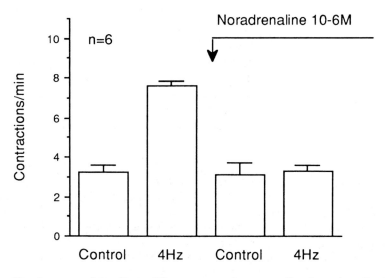

Figure 15. – Summary of the effects of *Ruscus* extract (upper panel) and noradrenaline (lower panel) on the mean lymphatic contraction frequency in response to field stimulation at 4Hz.

tion at 4 Hz, *Ruscus* extract caused it to be potentiated. This might suggest that *Ruscus* is acting on different receptors in these vessels from those through which noradrenaline is acting.

References

1. Aukland K, Nicolaysen G. Interstitial fluid volume : local regulatory mechanisms. Physiol Rev 1981; 61 : 556-643.
2. Guyton AC, Taylor AE, Granger HJ. *Circulatory Physiology II:Dynamics and control of the body fluids.* W.B. Saunders Compagny, Philadelphia, 1975.
3. Rusznyak I, Foldi M, Szabo G. *Lymphatics and Lymph Circulation.* Oxford : Pergamon Press 1967.
4. Yoffey JM, Courtice FC. *Lymphatics, lymph and the lymphomyeloid complex.* Academic Press, London. 1970.
5. Smith RO. Lymphatic contractility - a possible intrinsic mechanism of lymphatic vessels for the transport of lymph. 1949; J Exp Med 90 : 497-509.
6. McHale NG, Roddie IC. The effect of transmural pressure on pumping activity in isolated bovine lymphatic vessels. J Physiol 1976; 261 : 255-269.
7. McHale NG, Thornbury KD. A method for studying lymphatic pumping activity in conscious and anaesthetised sheep. J Physiol 1986; 378 : 109-118.
8. Zweifach BW, Prather JW. Micromanipulation of pressure in terminal lymphatics on the mesentery. Am J Physiol 1975; 228 : 1326-1335.
9. Reddy NP, Staub NC. Intrinsic propulsive activity of thoracic duct perfused in anaesthetised dogs. Microvasc Res 1981; 21 : 183-192.
10. Uhley HN, Leeds SE, Sampson JJ, *et al.* Role of pulmonary lymphatics in chronic pulmonary œdema. *Circ Res* 1962; 11 : 966-970.
11. Williamson IM. Some responses of bovine mesenteric arteries, veins and lymphatics. J Physiol 1969; 202 : 112-113P.
12. Johnston MG. Involvement of lymphatic collecting ducts in the physiology and pathophysiology of lymph flow. *In:Experimental biology of the lymphatic circulation,* MG Johnston ed., pp 81-120, Elsevier Science Publishers, B.V., 1985.
13. McHale NG, Roddie IC. The effect of intravenous adrenaline and noradrenaline infusion on peripheral lymph flow in the sheep. J Physiol 1983; 341 : 517-526.
14. McHale NG, Roddie IC. The effects of catecholamines on pumping activity in isolated bovine mesenteric lymphatics. J Physiol 1983; 338 : 527-536.
15. McHale NG, Roddie IC, Thornbury KD. Nervous modulation of spontaneous contraction in bovine mesenteric lymphatics. J Physiol 1980; 309 : 461-472.
16. McGeown JG, McHale NG, Thornbury KD. The effect of electrical stimulation of the sympathetic chain on popliteal efferent lymph flow in the anaesthetised sheep. J Physiol 1987; 393 : 123-133.
17. McCullough JS, McHale NG. Pressure flow relationships in isolated bovine mesenteric lymphatics during field stimulation. J Physiol 1988; 396 : 177P.

18. Allen JM, McCarron JG, McHale NG, *et al*. Release of Noradrenaline from the sympathetic nerves to bovine mesenteric lymphatic vessels and its modification by α-agonists and antagonists. Br J Pharmacol 1988; 94 : 823-833.

19. Su C, Bevan JA. The release of ^{3}H -norepinephrine in arterial strips studied by the technique of superfusion and transmural stimulation. J Pharmacol Exp Ther 1970; 172 : 62-68.

20. Allen JM, McCarron JG, McHale NG, *et al*. β-adrenoceptor mediated facilitation of noradrenaline release from the sympathetic nerves to bovine mesenteric lymphatic vessels. Br J Pharmacol 1989; 96 : 45-50.

21. Allen JM, McHale NG, Rooney BM. Effect of norepinephrine on contractility of isolated mesenteric lymphatics. Am J Physiol 1983; 244 : H479-H486.

22. Allen JM, Iggulden HLA, McHale NG. Beta-adrenergic inhibition of bovine mesenteric lymphatics. J Physiol 1986; 369 : 401-411.

23. McHale NG, Allen JM, Iggulden HLA. Mechanism of alpha-adrenergic excitation in bovine lymphatic smooth muscle. Am J Physiol 1987; 252 : H873-H884.

24. Sadoshima, Jun-Ichi, Akaike, *et al*. Cyclic AMP modulates Ca-activated K channel in cultured smooth muscle cells of rat aortas. Am J Physiol 1988; 255 : H754-H759.

25. McHale NG, Carl A, Sanders KM. Ca^{++} activated K$^+$ channels in canine lymphatic smooth muscle. Ir J Med Sci 1989; 158 : 130.

26. McHale NG, Allen JM, McCarron JG. Transient excitatory responses to sustained stimulation of intramural nerves in isolated bovine lymphatic vessels. Quart J Exp Physiol 1988; 73 : 175-182.

Return circulation and Norepinephrine : an update. Ed. P.M. Vanhoutte. John Libbey Eurotext, Paris © 1991, pp. 89-95

8

Effect of *Ruscus* extract on peripheral lymphatic vessel pressure and flow

G. Pouget, L. Ducros, G. Marcelon

Centre de Recherches Pierre Fabre, 17, avenue Jean Moulin, 81106 Castres-Cedex

Introduction

The sympathetic nervous system regulates the tone of the "Return Circulation"; under this name, we include the venules, veins and lymphatic vessels [9]. The role of lymphatic system is to remove the excess liquid (water, lipids, proteins,...) from the extracellular space and to conduct it to the heart.

In the periphery, the capture of lymph is ensured by an oncotic gradient, and the propulsion to the heart by lymphangion, small contractile units innervated by the adrenergic system [7]. It has been demonstrated that calcium-antagonists diminish or stop this "pumping system" and, in this sense, induced peripheral edema [6].

Ruscus extract, an alpha1- and alpha2-adrenergic agonist in veins [3], causes contractions *in vitro* and *in vivo* on the thoracic lymph duct [5]. Moreover, *Ruscus* enhances the spontaneous contractions of bovine mesenteric lymphatic vessels and potentiates the response to norepinephrine in these vessels [8].

The present study was designed, first, to demonstrate *in vivo* the effect of *Ruscus* on pressure and flow in a peripheral lymphatic vessel and, second, to determine whether or not this extract could counteract the edema-formation due to calcium-antagonists.

Material and methods

Experimental models

In anesthetized dogs (sodium pentobarbital 30 mg/kg), we isolated a lymph vessel which was parallel to the saphenous vein at the ankle level. All the lymph vessels were previously coloured by injection in the foot pad of 1 ml 1 % Evans Blue solution. After catheterization, other lymphatic vessels were ligated. The catheter was a polyethylene tube (Biotrol 113; external diameter 0.7 mm) which was connected to a pressure transducer (Sensortec, SCX 0.1D) and an electronic drop counter (Bret Electronique).

Determination of oncotic pressure

Next to the drop counter, samples of lymph were collected at 10 minute intervals. Ten microliters of lymph were diluted to 1 ml with saline solution and the absorbance of total proteins was measured at 280 nm with an UV-visible spectrophotometer (Beckman DU6)

The oncotic pressure (Ponc) was expressed, in water centimeter, as : Ponc = (Pt x 0.45) + (Pt x 0.078) where Pt was the concentration of total proteins in g/l.

Experimental protocols

— Determination of pressure and flow dose/response to *Ruscus:*a water-soluble extract of *Ruscus* was injected in the brachial vein at 1,2 and 5 mg/kg. These doses were chosen because they are venotonic in dogs [4].

— Determination of *Ruscus* activity after calcium antagonist injection : between two IV-injections of *Ruscus,* we injected nifedipine intravenously. The activity of *Ruscus* (5 mg/kg) was followed during one hour; then, nifedipine (0.1 mg/kg) during half an hour (we had previously verified that the activity of this dosis was maintained during more than one hour); finally, *Ruscus,* at the same dosis, during one more hour.

The flow was continuously monitored and the lymph was harvested at 10 minute intervals.

Results

Dose/response curve to *Ruscus*

During one hour after *Ruscus* injection, we observed the lymph pressure and flow. The first did not statistically vary in function of the dosis of the extract *(Figure 1)*. However, the flow was enhanced in duration and intensity in a

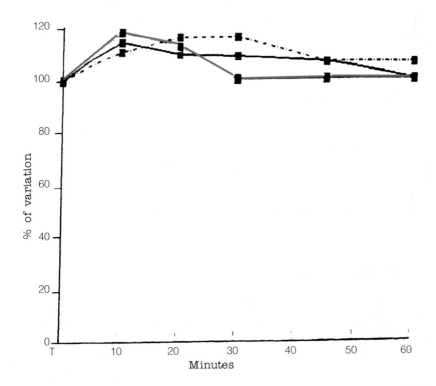

Figure 1. – Dose/response to *Ruscus* : % of variation of the lymphatic pressure in fonction of time after injection. (—■— 1 mg/kg, ---■--- 2 mg/kg, —■— 5 mg/kg).

dose-dependent way *(Figure 2)*; the area under the curve was statistically increased (p<0.01) at 2 and 5 mg/kg as compared to 1 mg/kg (5 dogs were used for each dosis).

Ruscus activity after nifedipine

As described above, *Ruscus* (5 mg/kg) augmented lymph flow after the first injection. At the same time, *Ruscus* enhanced the oncotic pressure in the circulatory lymph, demonstrating that *Ruscus* could extract the protein from the interstitial tissue.

When nifedipine was injected, the lymph flow diminished and the oncotic pressure fell slightly. The second *Ruscus* injection induced the same augmentation of lymph flow than the first one but a more pronounced enhancement of the oncotic pressure *(Figure 3)*.

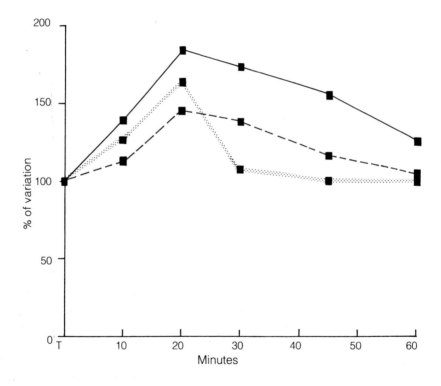

Figure 2. – Dose/response to *Ruscus:* % of variation of the lymph flow in fonction of time after injection. (—■— 1 mg/kg, ---■--- 2 mg/kg, —■— 5 mg/kg).

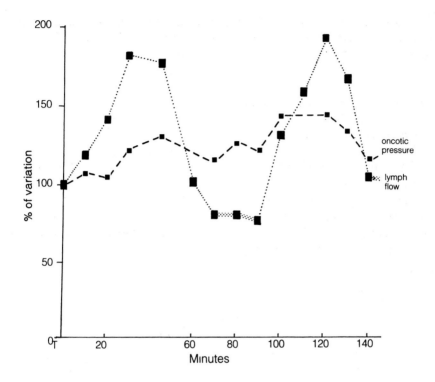

Figure 3. – Interactions *Ruscus* (5 mg/kg) and nifedipine (0.1 mg/kg)) on lymph flow and oncotic pressure.

Discussion

Ruscus extract, an alpha1- and alpha2-agonist, is a venotonic drug acting *in vitro* on the lymphatic system with the same mechanism of action [5]. *In vivo*, *Ruscus* is able to enhance the thoracic duct lymph flow, but its effect on the peripheral lymphatic system is unknown. To explore this system, we developed a model to study the small lymphatic vessel of the hindpaw of the dog. The dose/response activity obtained with *Ruscus* was in the same range as in the veins. The enhancement of the flow, in duration and intensity, without variation in pressure, reflected the augmentation of the contractility of lymph vessels as McHale had demonstrated *in vitro* on bovine mesenteric lymph vessels [8]. This rise in contractility corresponded to an enhancement of the "pumping system"; thus the propulsion of peripheral lymph toward the heart was more intense as also seen at the level of the thoracic duct [5].

In terms of edema, we had to remove not only liquid but also proteins. We have demonstrated that the oncotic pressure was augmented following *Ruscus* injection. In this sense, *Ruscus* could remove the inflammatory components of edema from the interstitial tissue. Moreover, at the microcirculatory level, Bouskela has demonstrated that *Ruscus* diminishes the permeability and enhances the venous flow without activity in arteries [1]. Altogether, these *Ruscus* activities favor a better return of blood and lymph from the legs to the heart.

The last part of the present study concerned the activity of *Ruscus* after injection of a calcium antagonist. The latter drugs enhance the microcirculatory permeability [1] and diminish the "pumping system" of lymph vessels [7]. It was of interest to know whether *Ruscus* could prevent these deleterious effects of calcium antagonists. The activity of *Ruscus* was unchanged after injection of nifedipine, demonstrating that the mechanism underlying the effect of *Ruscus* on peripheral lymphatics does not involve the opening of voltage operated calcium-channels.

In terms of its therapeutic effect in humans, *Ruscus* has been used to treat "heavy leg syndrome" at the microcirculatory, lymphatic and venous levels. Moreover, *Ruscus* can counteract the side effect of calcium antagonists during edema formation, as demonstrated in a clinical trial [2]. The present study indicates that these beneficial therapeutic effects of *Ruscus* can be attributed, at least in part, to a direct action on peripheral lymphatics.

References

1. Bouskela E. Microcirculatory responses in hamster cheek pouch to *Ruscus* extract. (In this issue).
2. Lagrue G, Behar A, Chaabane A, *et al.* Calcium antagonists induced edema. Effect of *Ruscus* extract on clinical and biological parameters. (In this issue).
3. Marcelon G, Verbeuren TJ, Lauressergues H, *et al.* Effect of *Ruscus aculeatus* on isolated canine saphenous veins. Gen Pharmacol 1983; 14 : 103-106.
4. Marcelon G, Lauressergues L, Vanhoutte PM. Mechanism of action of *Ruscus* extract : correlation between *in vitro* and *in vivo* studies. XIIIth world congress of the International union of angiology, Rochester (USA) 1983.
5. Marcelon G, Pouget G, Tisne-Versailles J. Effect of *Ruscus* extract on the adrenoceptors of the canine lymphatic thoracic duct. Phlebology 1988; 3 : Suppl. 1, 109-112.

6. McHale NG, Thornbury KD. A method for studying lymphatic pumping activity in conscious and anesthetized sheep. J Physiol 1986; 378 : 109-118.

7. McHale NG. Neural control of lymphatic pumping. Phlebology 1988; 3 : Suppl. 1, 105-108.

8. McHale NG. Mechanism of noradrenaline action in lymphatic vessels. (In this issue).

9. Shepherd JT, Vanhoutte PM. The human cardiovascular system. Facts and concepts. Raven Press, New York, 1979.

Return circulation and Norepinephrine : an update. Ed. P.M. Vanhoutte. John Libbey Eurotext, Paris © 1991, pp. 97-103.

9

Peripheral edema induced by calcium antagonists Interest of the ^{99m}Tc-albumin test to estimate an effect on capillary filtration

A. Behar, G. Lagrue, N. Bouarfa, A. Chaabane

Department of biophysic and nuclear medicine, Hôtel-Dieu, Paris, France

The calcium antagonists are a heterogenous group of drugs that possess both a negative inotropic effect on the heart and relaxation of vascular smooth muscle. These substances also cause clinically important peripheral edema as a side effect during treatment. With a ^{99m}Tc-albumin test, used to detect cyclic orthostatic edema [1], we have studied the effects of calcium antagonists on capillary filtration and in lymphatic resorption.

Twelve out-patients treated with calcium antagonists (nifedipine or nicardipine) suffering from evident edema, were treated also with *Ruscus* extract* (2 tablets per day) during a 28 to 40 days period.

---

* Cyclo-3 Fort®

Methodology

The test is carried out on the upper limbs by continually recording the injected radioactivity with a gamma-camera. The radioactive curve is measured at the forearm after the intravenous injection followed by a few minutes of tourniquet; the radioactivity then increases to a maximum.

In normal subjects, the radioactivity returns to the initial state in 3 min, and 10 min after the removal of the tourniquet it is identical to the initial values. The study of 420 files of female patients suffering from cyclic edema compared with a population of 100 normal women, showed that there always remained and additional residual radioactivity at 10 min which amounted to at least 8 % of the maximal value *(Figures 1)*.

A second phenomenon occurred after removal of the tourniquet : the curve was either smooth usually when the test was normal, or it presented irregular oscillations. In this case, the test was often pathological *(Figures 2 and 3)*.

To explain this phenomenon, the test was supplemented by a study involving double labelling using ^{131}I-albumin and ^{99m}Tc-red cells in ten healthy subjects and ten patients with untreated ICO. Evaluation of retention level after tourniquet release showed no retention of red cells in both populations and no albumin retention in the healthy subjects whilst it was pathological in ICO patients. The curve of decreasing radioactivity was often marked by irregular oscillations after removal of the tourniquet.

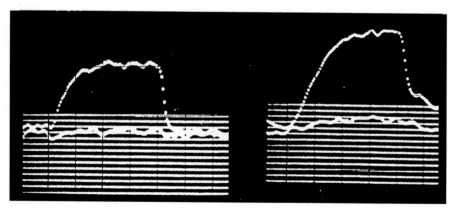

Figure 1. – Left : Normal test. Right : Cyclic edema. Example of continuous recording with gamma camera after radioactivity injection. Left : Normal subject. Right : Pathological subject.

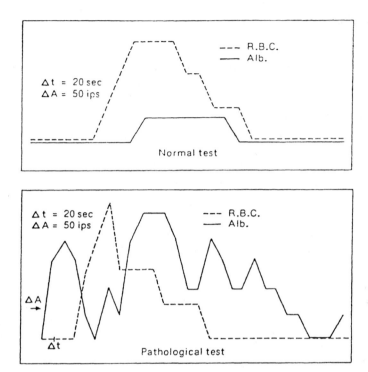

Figures 2 (top) and 3 (bottom). – After removal of the tourniquet the radioactivity curves were either smooth (Figure 2 : Normal test) or irregular (Figure 3 : Pathological test).

Study of these oscillations by fast fourier transformation (FFT) revealed reproductible abnormalities in the 37 to 20 mHz zone only in the ICO patients. Each point of the curve corresponds to the cumulative radioactivity over 10 sec for 25 min. This curve was then transformed into frequency diagram with the FFT function :

$$A_{(f)} = \int_{-\infty}^{+\infty} A(t) \exp. (-j2 \pi ft) \, dt.$$

(Voir Figure 4)

The abnormalities took the form of more frequent peaks with higher amplitudes than in the healthy subjects and were linked-in the case of excessive leak of albumin from capillaries to lymphatic resorption.

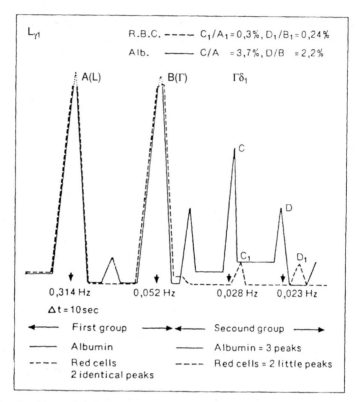

Figure 4. – Double test in idiopathic edema (FFT graph).

In the high frequency zone between 630 and 39 mHz, results corresponding to variations related to arteriovenous compliance were similar in both populations and by both tests.

An Open study in 15 patients with calcium antagonist treatment was carried out to study the pharmacodynamic activity of *Ruscus* extract. Fourteen patients had abnormal albumin retention and 12 had also, in the second low frequency zone, more than two peaks with a large relative amplitude ≥ 1 %.

Results

In these twelve patients, the mean retention of the labelled albumin was initially high : 14.5 %±4 %. With *Ruscus* extract all the test were normal, with a mean retention : 0.5 %±0.5 %.

The frequency diagram were abnormal. The mean number of peaks was initially : 4 peaks±1. After *Ruscus* extract treatment, the mean number of peaks was 2 peaks±1 (with 6 patients higher than 2 peaks, and 6 patients lower than 2 peaks).

Discussion

Taylor [5] proposed an original model of transcapillary filtration; he suggested that there was a transcapillary filtration of proteins, promoted by the negative pressure in the pericapillary space, and elective resorption of the protein excess by the lymphatic system. Our test is compatible with this model, because it reveals two abnormalities : excess filtration of albumin and the defect in lymphatic absorption. 14 out of 15 patients with calcium antagonists were in this case.

Edemas under calcium antagonists are not the result of a limb deficiency associated with a natrium and water retention, as suggested by the lack of resistance to diuretics, the non-increase of plasmatic volume and the lack of body weight-gain. They cannot be the result of an increased venous pressure due by cardiac abnormality either since there is no sign of cardiac insufficiency. Moreover, the hemodynamic studies do not show any evidence of a decrease in cardiac index. Finally, they cannot be due to decrease of plasmatic proteins concentration resulting of lower oncotic pressure.

Gustafsson [2] proposed a " comprehensive " physiopathological model : first, the vasodilatation produced by calcium antagonists led to an increased capillary hydrostatic pressure and thus to fluid filtration.

Second, these agents interfere with local vascular control in the tissue in turn leading to impaired autoregulation of hydrostatic pressure and impaired protection against the increased hydrostatic load.

But Gustafsson insists that the increase in hydrostatic pressure by calcium antagonist-induced vasodilatation was due to a relatively more pronounced decline in precapillary resistance (Ra) than in postcapillary resistance (Rv), leading to a decrease in Ra/Rv.

The calcium antagonists might cause a more pronounced dilatation of large arterial resistance vessels, leaving the small arteries (including precapillary sphincters) relatively unaffected. Thus, an increase in both arterial and venous pressures leads to a myogenic resetting of Ra/Rv counteracting the increase in hydrostatic pressure, and to a myogenic precapillary sphincter constriction, leading to a decrease in the capillary surface area available for fluid exchange. This would protect against outward filtration of intravascular fluid. The myogenic protection against increased hydrostatic load was inhibited by nifedipine in a dose-dependent way, thereby leading to edema occurring at a higher rate than normal. Third, fluid efflux normally exceeds influx across the capillary wall ; but the extra fluid enters the lymphatics and drains through them back into the blood.

The majority of authors agree on these three mechanisms but discuss the alterations of capillary filtration, found by Ohnmeiss and Nazzari [3] ; for example Gustaffson said : "Capillary filtration coefficient reflects alterations in the size of the perfused capillary surface area (as controlled by the activity of precapillary sphincters), and alterations in specific capillary permeability; thus, the effects of nifedipine on capillary filtration coefficient were small and not statistically significant even when the vasodilatation was pronounced". In the present study, the fact that 14 out of 15 patients exhibited an abnormal ^{99m}Tc-albumin test, suggest an evident alteration in capillary filtration for proteins (and of course for water).

This mechanism, probably, is very important to involved edema, like idiopathic cyclic edema situation. However, the contraction of lymphatic vessels plays an important role in regulating lymph flow. McHale [4] shows in 1983 the importance of the calcium concentration in spontaneous isometric contractions of isolated lymphatic vessels. Reduction in calcium concentration increased the frequency but decreased the force of the spontaneous contraction and ultimately abolished them.

The calcium antagonist decreased the force of spontaneous contractions without increasing their frequency. More over, the calcium ions are important for control of pacemaking (lymphatic pump), for propagation of the impulse and for the contractile response itself in these bovine lymph vessels.

Our test of capillary permeability confirms the excessive filtration of albumin in nifedipine-induced edema and the consequences on the frequency spectrum : the twelve patients suffering from nifedipine-induced edema presented more numerous peaks with considerably larger amplitude. These pulsatile effects suggest a distinct protein filtration during the arteriovenous load transport with phases of saturation and desaturation which may well support Taylor's hypothesis [5] of a "peripheral lymphatic heart".

It is now known that the lymphatic system carries out this function via the lymphatic pump presents in the capillary area. If the relaxation of lymphatic smooth muscle were induced by calcium antagonists, this would be a new mechanism for edema by saturation of the lymphatic draining of proteins.

In conclusion, this preliminary report suggests five mechanisms for edema induced by calcium antagonists :

— Vasodilatation with more dilatation of small arteries.

— Increased capillary hydrostatic pressure, by impaired capillary resistance.

— Increased lymph flow (but decreased lymphatic resorption of fluids).

— Excessive filtration of albumin.

— Decreased lymphatic draining of proteins by saturation of the lymphatic pump.

Ruscus is probably active in the last 3 mechanisms. A double blind placebo-controlled, randomised trial is underway to test in more details the pharmacodynamic activity of *Ruscus* extract.

References

1. Behar A, Lagrue G, Cohen-Boulakia F, *et al.* Capillary filtration idiopathic cyclic edema. Nuclear Medicine 1988; 27 : 105, 107.
2. Gustafsson D. Microvascular mechanisms involved in calcium antagonist edema formation. Journal of Cardiovascular Pharmacology 1987; 10 : (suppl. I) 121-131.
3. Ohnmeiss H, Nazzari M. Side effects of calcium antagonists. Am J Nephrol 1986; suppl. I, 81-86.
4. McHale NG, Allen JM. The effect of the external Ca^{2+} concentration on the contractility of bovine mesenteric lymphatics. Microvascular research 1983; 26, 2 : 182-192.
5. Taylor AE. Starling forces and lymph flow. Circulation research 1981; 49 : 557-575.
6. Chaabane A. Contribution à l'élaboration d'un modèle microcirculatoire pour les œdèmes induits par les inhibiteurs calciques. 1989; Thèse de médecine, Broussais-Hôtel-Dieu.

Return circulation and Norepinephrine : an update. Ed. P.M. Vanhoutte. John Libbey Eurotext, Paris © 1991, pp. 105-109.

10

Edema induced by calcium antagonists. Effects of *Ruscus* extract* on clinical and biological parameters

G Lagrue*, A Behar, A Chaabane**, J Laurent***

* Nephrology Department, Henri-Mondor Hospital, Créteil 94, France
** Biophysic Department, Broussais Hospital, Paris 14, France

During treatment with calcium antagonists edema of the ankles and legs is frequent, especially with dihydropyridines. The incidence varies from 3 to 60 % according to different authors [3, 5, 6]. The mechanism of this edema syndrome is unclear. It is not linked to renal troubles : water and sodium excretion are not decreased. Three factors appear involved.

• The precapillary arteriolar dilatation is predominant upon postcapillary venular dilatation, resulting in enhancement of hydrostatic intracapillary pressure, as suggested by Gustafsson [2].

• Capillary hyperpermeability to albumin and reduction in lymphatic pump activity are present, as demonstrated by Tc 99m albumin test and discussed in another chapter of this book (1).

• Capillary hyperpermeability to albumin and decreased lymphatic drainage are characteristic features of idiopathic orthostatic edema [4]. In this syndrome vasoactive substances such as *Ruscus* extract*, diosmine, flavonoids

---

* Cyclo-3 Fort®

are efficient to correct the capillary and lymphatic abnormalities, and simultaneous by induce clinical improvement [4]. This prompted us to study the clinical and biological effect of *Ruscus* extract + hesperidine methyl chalcone in hypertensive patients with calcium antagonist induced edema.

Methods

Eleven patients were studied (39-65 years old - median 56 years old): 6 men and 5 women. The clinical diagnosis was : essential hypertention (7 cases) hypertension secondary to glomerular nephropathy, with proteinuria, without any renal edema (4 cases); renal function was normal in all cases.

Edema of legs and ankles appeared during calcium-antagonist treatment by dihydropyridine derivatives (Nifedipine 40 mg/day and nicardipine 60 mg/day); headaches and facial flush were associated in 8 cases. The 99m Tc Albumin test as described by Behar [1] was performed before and after 6-8 weeks of treatment by *Ruscus* extract (three tablets a day; without modifying other treatments).

Results

Before treatment the Tc-Albumin test was abnormal in all patients *(Figures 1, 2)* with an enhanced capillary hypermeability to albumin with retention index from 8 % to 25 % (median 14 %) and an abnormal lymphatic resorption with 3-6 peaks (median 4).

After treatment the clinical results (9 patients) were assessed with a complete improvement observed in 4 patients with disappearance of edema and facial flush (the improvement was partial in 3 patients, and the edema was unchanged in 2 patients).

In all patients the blood pressure, which was well controlled by Ca-antagonists treatment remained at the initial levels. Tolerance was good without any side-effects. The biological abnormalities of the 99m-Tc albumin test were improved *(Figures 1, 2)* : the capillary hyperpermeability to albumin was normalized in the 11 cases, with a retention index < 1 % and the lymphatic resorption was normalized in 5 cases, improved in 2 cases and unchanged in 4 cases. Finally, the proteinuria initially present in 4 cases, decreased of 50 % in 3 cases, becoming null in 1 case.

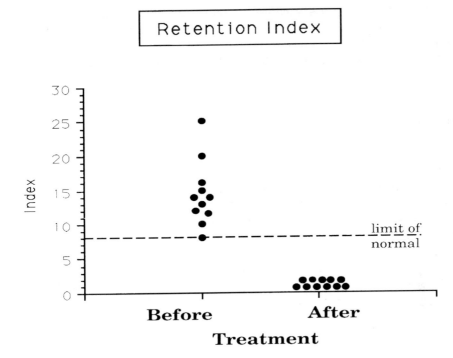

Figure 1. – Retention index of albumin before and after *Ruscus* extract treatment.

Discussion

These results indicate that Ca^{++}-antagonists-induced edema are linked, at least partly, to a capillary hyperpermeability to albumin, with an abnormal lymphatic resorption. These troubles are due to Ca-channel blockade, with reduction in myogenic (arteriolar and lymphatic) tone. During treatment with *Ruscus* extract, these biological abnormalities improved and simultaneously the edema disappeared or decreased in 7 out 9 cases.

The abnormal lymphatic resorption was not secondary to albumin excess concentration in interstitial fluid since lymphatic resorption remained abnormal in few cases even when capillary hyperpermeability to albumin had disappeared; thus abnormal lymphatic resorption was obviously linked to a functional defect in the lymphatic pump following an alteration of muscular tone of the lymphatic wall.

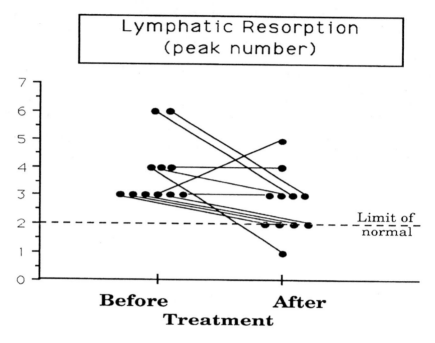

Figure 2. – Lymphatic resorption before and after *Ruscus* extract treatment.

Moreover reduction of proteinuria was observed in 3 out 4 cases. In hypertensive glomerular nephropathies it was recently demonstrated that conversion enzyme inhibitors (such as captopril) may decrease proteinuria; on the contrary, an enhanced proteinuria sometimes occurs with Ca-antagonists⁻ (such as nifedipine). As the *Ruscus* extract decreased the proteinuria, this suggests that the increase in proteinuriae associated with Ca^{++}-antagonists is linked to the drug-induced capillary hyperpermeability.

In summary, Ca^{++}-antagonists-evoked edema are an experimental model of capillary and lymphatic troubles, which is useful to study the action of vasoactive drugs.

References

1. Behar A, Lagrue G, Cohen-Boulakia F, *et al.* Capillary filtration in idiopathic cyclic edema. Nuclear Medecine 1988; 27 : 105-107.

2. Gustafsson D. Microvascular mechanisms involved in calcium antagonist edema formation. J Cardiovascular Pharmacology 1987; 10 (suppl. I) : 121-131.

3. Krebs R. Adverse reactions with calcium antagonists. Hypertension, 1983 ; 5 (suppl. III) : 125.

4. Lagrue G, Weil B, Behar A. Le syndrome d'œdèmes cycliques idiopathiques. J Mal Vasc 1977; 2 : 93-100.

5. Petru MA, Crawford MH, Sorensen SG *et al.* Short and long-term efficacy of high-dose oral diltiazem for angina due to coronary artery disease : a placebo-controlled, randomised, doble-blind crossover study. Circulation 1983; 68 : 139.

6. Schnapp P, Hermann H, Cernak P. Nifedipine monotherapy in the hypertensive elderly; a placebo-controlled study. Current Med Research Opinion 1987; 10 : 407-413.

Return circulation and Norepinephrine : an update. Ed. P.M. Vanhoutte. John Libbey Eurotext, Paris © 1991, pp. 111-119.

11

Therapeutic effect of *Ruscus* extract* in lymphedemas of the extremities

**J.A. Jimenez Cossio*, P.J. Magallon Ortin*,
M.T. Capilla Montes*, J. Coya Vina****

** Angiology and Vascular Surgery Service ; ** Nuclear Medicine Service,
Hospital "La Paz", Madrid, Spain*

Introduction

Lymphedema, defined as the accumulation of protein-rich interstitial fluid secondary to an alteration of the lymphatic system and generally located in the extremities, is a clinical entity that has been the subject of the attention of numerous clinical and basic research groups in recent times. Even though huge gaps remain in the knowledge of lymphatic pathology, new diagnostic techniques are appearing as a result of continued investigation into its physiopathological bases and drugs are available which, when associated with other means, improve lymphedema considerably.

The action of the current so-called lymphodrugs tends to cover all physiopathological aspects of the lymphedema, such as increase in the lymphatic debit, lymph formation and transport and protein mobilization. Upon acting on the α-adrenergic receptors located in the lymphatic wall, vasopressor agents could be capable of increasing lymphatic debit and transport. For

---

*Fabroven®

their part, benzopyrones and their derivatives could be capable of significantly increasing the number and activity of the macrophages and inducing a reduction in the high molecular weight proteins in the connective tissue, which are essential features of lymphedema treatment.

Ruscus aculeatus extract possesses a venotonic activity, widely demonstrated in pharmacology, through a direct action by stimulation of the postsynaptic $\alpha 1$ and $\alpha 2$-adrenergic receptors of the smooth muscle cell of the vein wall and by an indirect action through the release of noradrenaline stored in the presynaptic nerve terminals [1-5]. These actions of *Ruscus aculeatus* extract enhance the tone of the vein wall [6] and are reflected in the clinical practice in a proven and quantifiable efficacy in the treatment of venous insufficiency of the lower members [7-10].

The lymphatics have a noradrenergic innervation which is characterized by postsynaptic α-adrenergic and presynaptic α-adrenergic receptors which can modulate neurotransmitter release [11-5].

The importance of the lymphatic system, its physiology and its physiopathology and the mechanism of action of the *Ruscus aculeatus* extract at the level of the vein wall led to a search of a possible activity at lymphatic smooth muscle level and it was demonstrated that *Ruscus aculeatus* extract increases the contractility of the canine thoracic duct, as well as lymphatic flow [16].

Transposed to human pathology, these pharmacological results suggest that *Ruscus aculeatus* extract can improve lymphatic circulation and that it may be an effective lymphedema treatment. On the other hand all venous affections are usually accompanied by lymphatic insufficiency [17], so a dual action of *Ruscus aculeatus* extract, venotonic and lymphagogue, would be extremely interesting from a therapeutic standpoint.

For its part, hesperidin methyl-chalcone, a benzopyronic derivative, increases the proteolytic capacity of macrophages and therefore reduces interstitial oncotic pressure, a fundamental component of edema. In addition, hesperidin methyl-chalcone reduces capillary permeability [18-20].

From the theoretical and pharmacological viewpoint the association of *Ruscus aculeatus* extract and hesperidin methyl-chalcone could be an association of high therapeutic efficacy in the treatment of lymphedema which will successfully increase lymphatic debit and reduce high molecular weight proteins in the interstitial tissue.

The objective of this study is to evaluate the therapeutic effect of *Ruscus* extract, both objectively and subjectively, on edemas of lymphatic etiology.

Material and methods

We admitted 12 patients (11 females and 1 male) to the study with ages ranging from 15 to 59 years (average 38.3).

They all exhibited lymphedema of the extremities : postmastectomy in 3 cases, hereditary (Milroy's disease) in 1 case and idiopathic in the other 8 cases. In total, 16 pathological extremities, 3 upper and 13 lower, were studied. The lymphedema evolution time was variable, ranging from 2 months to 29 years (average 7.05).

The symptoms exhibited were edema (100 % of cases), sensation of tension (100 % of cases) and pain (66.6 % of cases).

The exclusion criteria were as follows :

• Pregnancy, postpartum

• Age below 10 years and above 60 years

• Active gastroduodenal ulcer

• Lymphangitis

• Renal or hepatic insufficiency

• Severe diseases

• Lack of cooperation

• Discontinuation of treatment in the course of the study

The patients were treated during a period of 2 months with orally administered *Ruscus* extract* in the form of drinkable ampoules, according to the following therapeutic schedule :

— 1st week : 6 ampoules a day (2-2-2) corresponding to 180 mg of *Ruscus aculeatus* extract and 900 mg of hesperidin methyl-chalcone.

— Weeks 2 to 8 : 4 ampoules a day (2-2-0) corresponding to 120 mg of *Ruscus aculeatus* extract and 600 mg of hesperidin methyl-chalcone.

All types of supplementary therapeutic measures (medication, hygienic and dietetic measures, compression) were discontinued two weeks before the start of treatment. The therapeutic efficacy evaluation criteria were the clinical symptoms, volume of the extremity and isotopic lymphography. The symptoms evaluated were pain, sensation of tension and heaviness. The intensity of the symptoms was rated by the patient on a scale of 0 to 3 : 0-absent, 1-mild, 2-moderate, 3-severe.

---

* 1 ampoule of Fabroven® = 30 mg of *Ruscus aculeatus* extract + 150 mg of hesperidin methyl-chalcone

The volume of the extremity was determined by Volometer® (Bösl Medizin-tecnick-Aachen, Germany), which provides an optoelectronic automatic volumetric measurement (mean error ± 0.5 %). The measurements were taken at the same time and after 15 minutes' decubital rest.

The lymphatic dynamics study was carried out by means of isotopic lymphography with colloid particles marked with 99m-Tc with a diameter between 2 and 20 nm. A dose of 1 to 3 mCi in a volume not exceeding 0.03-0.1 ml was injected subcutaneously at the level of the 1st and 2nd interdigital spaces of both extremities. Body scanning was then carried out. Gamma camera images were obtained at 10, 30, 60, 90, 120 and 240 minutes and the morphology of the lymphatic system was evaluated from the feet to the abdomen, including the inguinal and axillary ganglia, the arrival time thereat and the rate of disappearance of the deposit.

The patients were seen prior to starting the treatment and after 4 and 8 weeks' treatment. An evaluation of each symptom was carried out at the first visit with the respective score. The volume of both extremities (upper or lower) was measured and isotopic lymphography was performed. The symptomatology was evaluated again after four weeks, the volume of the extremities was determined and possible side effects of the treatment were investigated, as well as any event that might affect the study. The determinations, including isotopic lymphography, were repeated at 8 weeks' treatment.

For statistical analysis we used the Student t-test for comparison of the two means and all type I (alpha) error probability less than 0.05 was considered statistically significant.

Results

The results were analysed separately for each criterion evaluated : symptomatology, volumetry, isotopic lymphography.

As regards symptomatology, after 8 weeks' treatment we observed a statistically significant improvement in each of the 3 symptoms evaluated *(Table I)*. Considering a major improvement to be any score that drops by two points, a clear improvement one that decreases by one point, and no improvement every score that remains unchanged, the 3 symptoms evaluated improved in the majority of the patients *(Figure 1)*. No deterioration was detected in any case.

Volumetry revealed a reduction in the edema in 81 % of the cases. After 8 weeks' treatment we detected an average decrease of 224.94 ml

Table I. – Trends in the scores (x±2 SD) corresponding to each of the symptoms evaluated.

Symptom	T0 week	T4 weeks	T8 weeks
Heaviness (n=12)	1,83±0,35	1,08±0,4*	0,58±0,35**
Pain (n=8)	1,38±0,56	0,75±0,53	0,63±0,39*
Tension (n=12)	1,75±0,27	1,17±0,43*	0,58±0,4*

*p<0.05, **p<0.001 (vs T0 weeks)

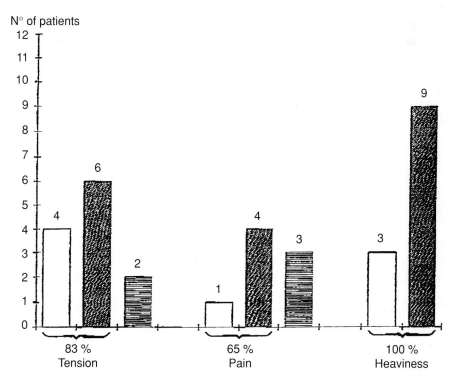

Figure 1. – Patients who improve for each of the symptoms evaluated.. ☐ Major improvement. ▨ Clear improvement. ▤ No improvement.

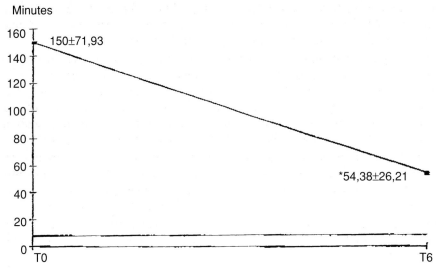

Figure 2. – Evolution of marked particle arrival time at the inguinal/axillary ganglia (x±2SD).
———— Pathological extremities
•———— Normal extremities
(*$p<0.05$ vs T0)

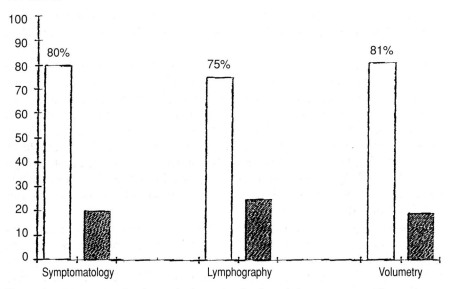

Figure 3. – Percentage of patients who improve after 8 weeks' treatment according to the parameter evaluated. ☐ Improvement. ▨ Unchanged.

(To : 2,590.94±191.67 - T8=2,366±254.88) without this difference being significant. At the end of the study we detected an increase in the edema, which was always less than 50 ml, in 19 % of the cases.

The isotopic lymphography was pathological in all cases and evident abnormalities were detected in three extremities which did not exhibit any symptom clinically. The marked particle arrival time at the inguinal/axillary ganglia in the pathological extremities was 150±71.93 versus the 5 minutes of normal extremities. After 8 weeks' treatment it dropped to approximately a third : 54.38±26.21. This difference is statistically significant *(Figure 2)*.

Globally, the three parameters evaluated improved after 8 weeks' treatment. The symptomatology improves in 80 % of the patients. The volumetry improves in 81 % of the cases and the isotopic lymphography shows an increase in the rate of lymphatic flow in 75 % of the cases *(Figure 3)*.

Insofar as tolerance is concerned, it was good and no major side effect was detected, so that it was not necessary to discontinue the treatment in any case.

Discussion

Although on a small group of patients, these results suggest that the association of *Ruscus aculeatus* and hesperidin methyl-chalcone is an effective treatment for lymphedema.

The three symptoms evaluated underwent considerable improvement. The sensation of heaviness and tension improved significantly already after the first four weeks' treatment and this improvement was consolidated during the following four weeks. In the case of pain, which was the least common symptom, although an improvement was already observed four weeks after the outset of treatment, it was necessary to wait until 8 weeks for this to be significant. Bearing in mind the evolutive tendency of the symptomatology associated with lymphedemas as well as their impact on the patient's life, these results show the beneficial nature of *Ruscus* extract, which acts uniformly on the three symptoms studied.

The volumetry performed with the Volometer®, a high precision, easily operated measuring instrument well accepted by the patient on account of the speed of the exploration and the absence of uncomfortable effects, revealed a reduction in volume of the extremities of 8.7 %, without this difference being significant. If we remember that lymphedema is a pathology of lengthy evolution which tends to worsen, these results are of interest and allow us to presume that *Ruscus* extract associated with other conservative measures (hygienic and dietetic measures, pressotherapy, lymphatic massage) in long term treatment will lead to considerable reduction in the edema.

Isotopic lymphography made it possible to confirm the diagnosis and carry out a dynamic study, which showed an increase in lymphatic flow after 8 weeks' treatment with *Ruscus* extract. The radioactive marker progression time from the point of injection to the inguinal/axillary ganglia fell by 63.7 % and an increase in lymphatic drainage was exhibited.

We also visualized an increase in the diversion of lymphatic flow through the trunks and a boosting of the transdermic superficial ones when the former are occluded. Overall, the data obtained with isotopic lymphography reveal an improvement of lymphatic function.

In conclusion, treatment with *Ruscus* extract improved the three parameters evaluated (symptomatology, volumetry, isotopic lymphography). These appreciable results were obtained with *Ruscus* extract as the only treatment, although pharmacological treatment is a partial aspect of global lymphedema therapeutics, which also includes hygienic and dietetic measures, pressotherapy, lymphatic massage. Despite the need for studies in larger series of patients, in long term and in association with other therapeutic measures, *Ruscus* extract appears to be a good therapeutic option in the treatment of lymphedema, a pathology where the therapeutic results are unspectacular and short-lived.

References

1. Marcelon G, Verbeuren TJ, Lauressergues H, *et al.* Effect of *Ruscus aculeatus* on isolated canine cutaneous veins. Gen Pharmac 1983; 14 : 103-106.

2. Marcelon G, Vanhoutte PM. Mechanism of action of *Ruscus* extract. Inter Angio 1984; 3 : 74-76,

3. Rubanyi G, Marcelon G, Vanhoutte PM. Effect of temperature on the responsiveness of cutaneous veins to the extract of *Ruscus aculeatus*. Gen Pharmac 1984; 15 : 431-434.

4. Branco D, Osswald W. The influence of *Ruscus* extract on the uptake and metabolism of noradrenaline in the normal and varicose human saphenous vein. Phlebology 1988 ; 3, suppl. 1 : 33-39.

5. Marcelon G, Vanhoutte PM. Venotonic effect of *Ruscus* under variable temperature conditions *in vitro*. Phlebology 1988; 3, suppl. 1 : 51-54.

6. Lauressergues H, Vilain P. Pharmacological activities of *Ruscus* extract on venous smooth muscle. Inter Angio 1984; 3 : 70-73.

7. Demarez JP, Laurent D. European validation of phlebotonic : a summary of French clinical studies demonstrating the activity of Cyclo 3. Phlebology 1988; 3, suppl. 1 : 133-138.

8. Sentou Y, Bernard-Fernier MF, Demarez JP, *et al.* Symptomatologie et plétysmographie : parallélisme des résultats obtenus lors d'un traitement par Cyclo 3 de patientes porteuses d'une insuffisance veineuse chronique. Gaz Med Fr 1985; 92 : 73-77.

9. Elbaz C, Nebot F, Reinharel D. Insuffisance veineuse des membres inférieurs. Etude contrôlée de l'action du Cyclo 3. Phlébologie 1976; 29 : 77-84.

10. Lozes A, Boccalaon H. Double blind study of *Ruscus* extract : venous plethysmographic results in man. Inter Angio 1984; 3 : 99-102.

11. Allen JM, McHale NG, Rooney AM. Effect of norepinephrine on contractility of isolated mesenteric lymphatics. Am J Physiol 1983; 244 : 479.

12. McHale NG, Roddie IC, Thornbury KD. Nervous modulation of spontaneous contractions in bovine mesenteric lymphatics. J Physiol 1980; 309 : 461.

13. Allen JM, McHale NG. Neuromuscular transmission in bovine mesenteric lymphatics. Microvasc Res 1986; 31 : 77-83.

14. Alessandrini C, Gerci R, Sacchi G *et al.* Cholinergic and adrenergic innervation of mesenterial lymph vessels in guinea pig. Lymphology 1981; 14 : 1-6.

15. McHale NG. Neural control of lymphatic pumping. Phlebology 1988; 3, suppl. 1 : 105-108.

16. Marcelon G, Pouget G, Tisne-Versailles J. Effect of *Ruscus* on the adrenoceptors of the canine lymphatic thoracic duct. Phlebology 1988; 3, suppl. 1 : 109-112.

17. Jimenez Cossio JA. Los linfáticos en la insuficiencia venosa crónica. *In:Progresos en linfologia.* Madrid, Jarpyo eds, 1987; 53-57.

18. Estler CJ. Zur pharmakologie der Bioflavonoide. Fortschr Med 1971; 89,16 : 669-671.

19. Tarayre JP, Lauressergues H. Preuves pharmacologiques de l'activité de l'héspéridine méthyl-chalcone. Angiologie 1975; 27 : 197-203.

20. Felix W, Schmidt G, Nieberce J. Protective effect of *Ruscus* extract against injury of vascular endothelium and vascular smooth muscle caused by ethacrymic acid. Inter Angio 1984; 3 : 77-79.

Return circulation and Norepinephrine : an update. Ed. P.M. Vanhoutte. John Libbey Eurotext, Paris © 1991, pp. 121-130.

12

Efficacy of *Ruscus* extract* in venolymphatic edema using foot volumetry

G. Rudofsky

Angiology Clinic and Policlinic, Essen University, Hufelandstraße 55, 4300 Essen 1, Germany

Edema-protective and α-adrenergic drugs could be used to support physiotherapy in venolymphatic edema, especially in the early stage of the disease, the aim being to increase the lymphatic load and also the tone of the blood vessels, thus increasing their pump performance and the pump function of the lymphatic vessels.

As a rule treatment is monitored by measuring the volume change in the edematous extremity, but without determining whether any such change concerns the tissue, the blood, or both. However, since vasoactive substances can alter the volume of the extremity both by reducing the storable blood volume and by edema protection and lymphokinetic effects, the efficacy of an antiedemic drug can only be demonstrated if one can differentiate between a change in blood volume and a change in tissue volume.

The therapeutically active constituents are *Ruscus* extract and trimethylhesperidin chalcone (TMHC) capsules. Both these substances have been shown to decrease capillary permeability in animal studies [1, 2]. In addition, the α-

---

* Phlebodril®

adrenergic active substances of the *Ruscus* extract cause venous constriction [3, 4]. This drug combination thus meets the requirement for a treatment for venolymphatic edema.

The capillary-sealing action has been confirmed in clinical studies on healthy volunteers subjected to pressure loading during plethysmography [5, 6]. Two randomized double-blind studies were performed to clarify the way in which edemas are reduced under the normal orthostatic conditions. The first of these studies investigated the effect of a single dose on the change in tissue and blood volumes. The second study aimed to determine the effect of long-term therapy.

Methods and patients

A technique which allows appropriate differentiation between blood and tissue volume was developed for volumetry of the foot and ankle region [7] *(Figure 1)*. The volume is first determined while the subject is in a standing position (foot volume). The measurement is then repeated while the extremity is largely empty of blood. The latter measurement can be regarded as the tissue volume and the difference between this and the first measurement represents the blood volume storable during orthostasis. This method is sensitive enough to register a loading-determined tendency towards swelling in the course of a day. It can thus be shown that in patients with chronic venous insufficiency caused by primary varicosis the increase in foot volume in the course of a day is essentially due to an increase in tissue volume, whereas there is no clear increase in the already elevated venous blood volume. In contrast, healthy volunteers show a significant increase in blood volume in the course of the day [7].

In the first randomized double-blind crossover study 20 healthy volunteers (11 men and 9 women aged between 20 and 43) took 450 mg *Ruscus* extract, 450 mg TMHC, 900 mg of a combination of the two substances, or a placebo as a single dose immediately before the first measurement. The volunteers were assigned to the four treatment groups on the basis of a randomization key. A 1-week washout phase was provided between the treatments.

To investigate the long-term effect, 141 patients (43 men and 98 women) with chronic venous insufficiency (CVI) were recruited to a randomized, double-blind, multicenter study. The cause of the CVI was either primary varicosis (81 patients) or post-thrombotic syndrome (PTS) (60 patients). After a 2-week washout the patients were given 4 weeks of treatment with 3 x 2

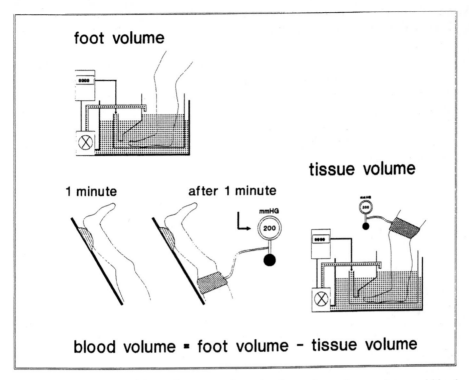

Figure 1. – Technique of foot volumetry to determine foot volume, tissue volume and blood volume.

and then 8 weeks of treatment with 2 x 2 capsules of *Ruscus* extract or placebo. The patients venous pump function during toe-stand exercises was also investigated plethysmographically [8].

Results

In healthy subjects both active substances significantly reduced the tissue volume (p < 0.01), although the effect of the *Ruscus* extract was about 3 times stronger than that of TMHC *(Figure 2)*. The two substances also showed different effects in respect of the storable blood volume. Owing to its

123

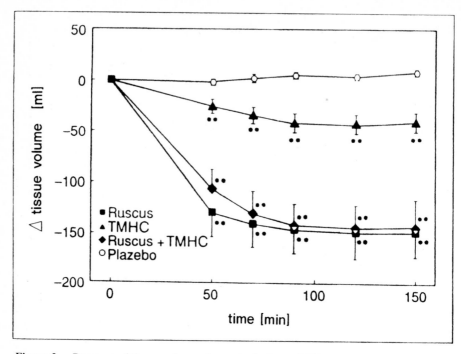

Figure 2. – Decrease of tissue volume after a single dose of 450 mg *Ruscus* extract, 450 mg trimethylhesperidin chalcone or the drug combination in healthy volunteers. ••: Significant difference compared to placebo (p<0.01).

vasoconstrictor properties, the *Ruscus* extract produced a decrease in the storable blood volume. After TMHC, however, the orthostatic blood volume of the healthy subjects increased *(Figure 3)*. The active substance combination of both substances produced blood volume changes which were between those determined for *Ruscus* extract and TMHC.

In the CVI patients there was a continuous decrease in the foot and ankle volume during the 12-week treatment with active substance. Under placebo, on the other hand, the foot volume showed a continuous increase caused by rising of the seasonal temperature. At the end of the study the volume difference between the active substance and the placebo was 65 ml in PTS patients and 47 ml in varicosis patients. In PTS patients, the tissue volume was reduced by the same degree as the foot volume *(Figure 4)*. The volume of

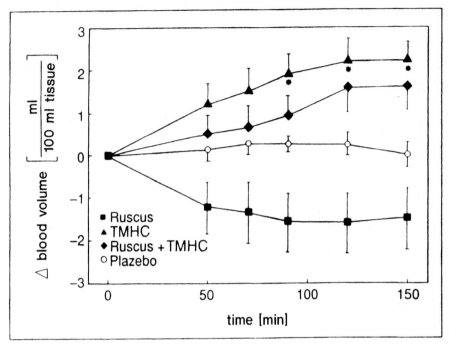

Figure 3. – Effect of *Ruscus* extract, trimethylhesperidin chalcone and the combination on blood volume of ankle region in healthy volunteers. ●: Significant difference compared to placebo (p<0.05).

blood stored in the ankle region during orthostasis was not affected by the medication.

Ruscus extract produced a significant reduction in leg swelling in varicosis patients too *(Figure 4)* (p < 0.05). However, this reduction is not due entirely to a decrease in tissue volume. The volume of blood stored in the veins during orthostasis was also significantly reduced. The reduction in blood volume accounts for about 11 % of the decrease in the foot volume.

Increasing the venous tone not only reduced the blood volume, it also brought about a considerable improvement in venous pump performance. After *Ruscus* extract capsules the volume of blood that could be pumped off with toe-stand exercises increased by 7 %, whereas in the placebo group the pump performance fell by 22 % *(Figure 5)*

125

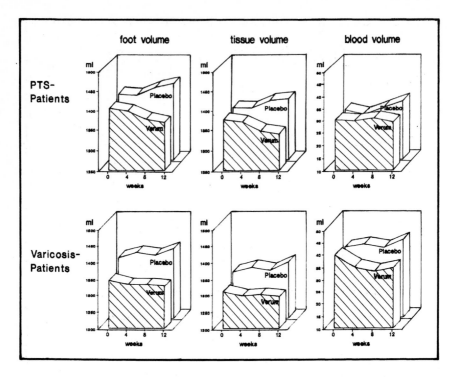

Figure 4. – Changes of foot, tissue and blood volume during the 12 weeks lasting treatment period in patients with chronic venous insufficiency caused by a postthrombotic syndrome or primary varicosis.

Discussion

In healthy subjects *Ruscus* extract produced a greater decrease than TMHC in the tissue volume. A possible explanation for the different behaviour of the two substances may be that the capillary-sealing action of TMHC reduced only the lymphatic load, causing the tissue volume to decrease to some extent. As Marcelon *et al.* [9] have shown, the α-adrenergic action of *Ruscus* extract increases the pump performance of the lymph vessels, thus also increasing lymph flow. The greater decrease in tissue volume under *Ruscus* extract could be the result of tissue volume reduction via increased lymphatic drainage as well as the capillary-sealing action. The improvement in venous

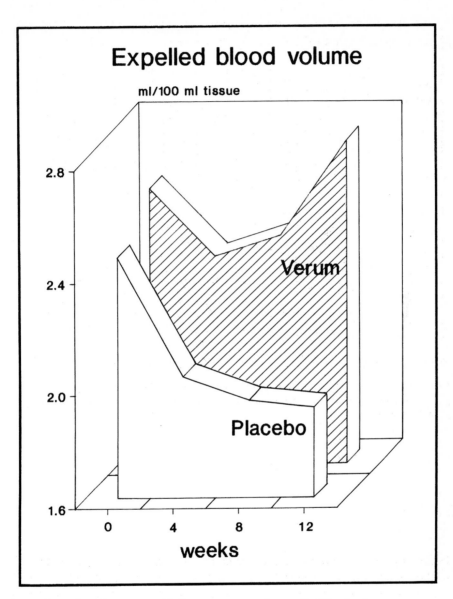

Figure 5. – Effect of treatment with *Ruscus* extract on the expelled blood volume.

pump function, such as was seen in patients with chronic venous insufficiency in primary varicosis in the multicenter study may also play an important role, since the volume of blood that can be pumped off correlates very

closely with venous pressure and thus corresponds to a decrease in filtration pressure in the capillary system.

The α-adrenergic action of *Ruscus* extract should also be regarded as a cause of the different effects on storable blood volume displayed by the two test substances. Owing to its vasoconstrictor properties, *Ruscus* extract produced a decrease in the storable blood volume. The increase under TMHC in healthy subjects should be seen as the result of reduced tissue pressure on the venous system, produced by a falling filtration rate and the associated drying-out of tissue, so that the veins are able to expand further and fill with blood. After *Ruscus* extract the increase in venous tone works against such expansion. The changes seen after the combination of active substance, therefore, were somewhere between the values determined for *Ruscus* extract and for TMHC.

An overlapping of the effects of *Ruscus* extract and TMHC on blood volume in patients can be ruled out, as the increased fluid content of the tissues is first normalized by the capillary-sealing action of TMHC. The relative drying-out compared to the normal state, which was observed in healthy subjects, does not occur. Dilation of the large-volume veins in varicosis patients was therefore not to be expected.

The changes in tissue and blood volume produced by long-term therapy differed according to the cause of the disease. In PTS patients the mean difference between the decreases in foot volume and tissue volume was less than 1 ml. In PTS patients, therefore, the significant reduction in the foot volume can be clearly attributed to a significant decrease in edema volume in the foot and ankle region. In contrast to the varicosis patients, however, blood volume was not affected. This seemingly contradictory behaviour of the two groups can be explained by the aetiology. Where there is impaired drainage of blood in the deep vein system, but otherwise intact vein systems, edema formation is at first in the foreground, since the veins do not yet show any pathological dilation (e.g. primary varicosis). Only when chronic blood volume overloading causes dilation of the veins serving as collateral drainage channels can one also expect an increase in venous capacity. However, such patients are then at a more severe stage of chronic venous insufficiency than those investigated here.

The tissue volume change of 45-60 ml (varicosis patients/PTS patients) corresponds to the edema increase measured in the absence of medication in CVI patients in the course of a day [7]. The loading-dependent tendency to swelling, which represents an important cause of subjective symptoms in patients with CVI, can therefore to a large extent be prevented by treatment with *Ruscus* extract and TMHC.

The continuous decrease in foot volume over the duration of the study shows that we are here dealing with slow reparative processes in the venous system which were still not concluded by the end of the study. Studies on patients who had to have the great saphenous vein removed provide an indication of what these processes are. They showed that with preoperative administration of *Ruscus* extract and TMHC there is a change in the activity of lysosomal enzymes and an increase in the fibrinolytic activity of the venous wall [10, 11]. Furthermore, long-term treatment with flavonoids stimulates the macrophages, increasing proteolysis of the edema protein in the interstitium. This ultimately leads to a reduction in edema [12]. Long-term therapy could therefore considerably reduce the progression of the venous disease or even bring it to a halt.

Together with the results from animal experiments and clinical studies, differential volumetry allows the establishment of an individual action profile for each constituent of *Ruscus* extract. The *Ruscus* extract/TMHC combination thus fulfills two requirements of a venous therapeutic agent for the treatment of chronic venous insufficiency : the capillary-sealing action of TMHC produces a clear reduction in edema volume, and an improvement in the associated subjective complaints : the venoconstrictor activity of *Ruscus* extract may accelerate the flow of blood and may reduce its viscosity. Venous stasis, and probably also the associated risk of thrombosis, may be thus opposed.

References

1. Felix W, Nieberle J, Schmidt G. Protektive Wirkung von Trimethylhesperidinchalkon und *Ruscus aculeatus* gegenüber dem Etacrynsäureödem an Hinterlauf der Katze. Phlebol und Proktol 1983; 12 : 209-218.
2. Hönig I. Effect of the permeability of the isolated ear vein of the pig ; a comparison between flavonoids and saponins. *In : Phlebologie 89*, A. Davy, R. Stemmer eds, 1989 John Libbey Eurotext Ltd, pp. 680-682.
3. Marcelon G, Vanhoutte PM. Venotonic effect of *Ruscus* under variable temperature conditions *in vitro*. Phlebology 1988; 3 (Suppl. 1) : 51-54.
4. Flavahan NA. Vanhoutte PM. Thermosensitivity of cutaneous and deep veins. Phlebology 1988; 3 suppl. 1 : 41-45.
5. Rudofsky G, Nobbe F. Zur Wirkung eines Kombinationspräparates auf die Venenkapazität. Fortschr Med 1982; 25 : 1217-1220.
6. Rudofsky G, Hirche H. Plethysmographische Untersuchungen eines Venentherapeutikums bei wärmebedingten hämodynamischen Veränderungen. Med Welt 1985; 36 : 145-149.
7. Rudofsky G, Bürkle S, Meyer P. Eine modifizierte Volumetrie zur Erfassung on intra- und extravasalen Volumina an der unteren extremität. *In :* Häring, R. (Ed.) : Berichtsband der

5 gemeinsamen Jahrestagung der Angiologischen Gesellschaften der BRD, Ôsterreichs und der Schweiz. R. 114 : 431-432 (1985), Demeter, Gräfelfing, 1986.

8. Rudofsky G, Diehm C, Gruß JD, *et al.* Chronisch venöse Insuffizienz : Behandlung mit *Ruscus*-Extrakt und Trimethylhesperidinchalkon. MMW 1990; 13 (Jahrg. 132) : 205-210.

9. Marcelon G, Pouget G, Tisné-Versailles J. Effect of *Ruscus* on the adrenoceptors of canine lymphatic thoracic duct. Phlebology 1988; 3 (Suppl. 1) : 109-112.

10. Seydewitz V. Biochemical investigations on the action of *Ruscus* extract and Trimethyl-hesperidinchalkon (TMHC). 3rd International Symposium : Return circulation and Nore-pinephrine : and update Cairo, March 12-16, 1990.

11. Haas S, Lill G. Effect of Phlebodril on the fibrinolytic activity of varicose veins. 3rd International Symposium : Return circulation and Norepinephrine : an update Cairo. March 12-16, 1990.

12. Casley-Smith JR. High protein edemas and the benzopyrones. Lippencott, Sydney, 1986.

Return circulation and Norepinephrine : an update. Ed. P.M. Vanhoutte. John Libbey Eurotext, Paris © 1991, pp. 131-137.

13

Changes induced by ageing and denervation in the canine saphenous vein ; a comparison with the human varicose vein

I. Azevedo, A. Albino Teixeira, W. Osswald

*Laboratório de Farmacologia, Faculdade de Medicina,
4200 Porto, Portugal*

Introduction

The varicose vein shows a number of changes which have been studied and described over the years, in careful descriptions of the morphological alterations characterizing varicose transformation of veins [1]. Proeminent changes consist in the greater thickness of the vein wall, increase in extracellular material, fibrosis and breakup of the cellular pattern ; the corresponding functional alteration dominating the picture being loss of distensibility.

We have been impressed by the fact that sympathetic denervation of the canine saphenous vein induces marked morphological changes of the vessel, some of them reminding us of the changes due to varicose transformation. The saphenous vein of the dog, deprived (by surgery or by intravenous administration of the selective neurotoxin 6-hydroxydopamine) of its sympathetic nerve supply, shows a marked thickening of the vessel wall, due to hypertrophy of the smooth muscle cells and increase in extracellular material, as well as a number of cellular and nuclear changes, as described earlier [2, 3]. In good agreement with these data, Dimitriadou *et al.* [4] described the same morphological alterations in arterial vessels of the rabbit, after surgical denervation.

The morphological alterations caused at the extraneuronal level by denervation of blood vessels were accompanied by a marked reduction in the ability of the tissue to metabolically handle noradrenaline and isoprenaline [2].

In our studies on normal and varicose human veins we found a number of similarities between the human varicose vein and the denervated canine vein, not only concerning the morphology but also the function of the noradrenaline metabolizing systems [5]. In fact, the varicose vein had a lower noradrenaline content than the normal vein and, when incubated with 3H-noradrenaline, accumulated and metabolized much less noradrenaline than its normal counterpart.

Therefore, it seemed of interest to further compare the normal and the varicose vein and to compare them with normal and denervated canine veins, using animals of different ages in order to obtain data concerning the effects of ageing on the vessel and its susceptibility to surgical denervation.

Material and methods

Segments of human saphenous veins were obtained at surgery (either from patients subjected to coronary bypass operations - normal veins, or from those undergoing operations for varicose veins - varicose veins). The segments were immediately washed in oxygenated, ice-cold Krebs-Henseleit fluid and transported to the laboratory; the interval between surgery and experimental procedure was never longer than 1 h.

Dog saphenous veins were obtained from mongrel animals anaesthetized with sodium pentobarbitone (30 mg/kg, i.v. injected in the forelimb) and prepared as described above. The dogs used were grouped, according to their age (established with the help of an independent veterinarian) in 3 groups : young (4 months to 1 year of age), mature (3 to 6 years of age) and old (7 years old and more) animals. In order to obtain denervation of the saphenous vein, the right lateral saphenous vein was exposed and carefully prepared under sterile conditions by blunt dissection, separating it from the surrounding connective tissue. Denervation was effected by applying artery clamps to the dorsal and plantar branches, just before their reunion to form the lateral saphenous vein, as well as to the main trunk of this vein, about 5 cm upstream. The calcaneal tributary, which is the only one of significant dimensions to enter the vein in this segment, was also clamped. Any other small tributaries were ligated. After 5 min, the clamps were released. The surgical wounds were closed with silk stitches and the dogs kept warm until they recovered from anaesthesia. One million units of clemizole-penicillin were injected i.m.; no wound infections were observed. The dogs were re-operated, under pentobarbital anaesthesia, 5 days later and segments of both denervated and control veins removed.

Noradrenaline content in the venous tissue was determined by HPLC-ED as described before [2]. The remaining venous tissue was used for morphological studies, using the methods previously described [2, 6-8].

Autoradiographic studies were done on human venous tissue sections after incubation with 0.1µmol/l of 3H-noradrenaline; for details see Azevedo and Osswald [9].

Human veins

The morphology of the human varicose vein differed substantially from that of the normal vein. The data obtained in sections from varicose veins (number of patients=8) showed, when compared with those of normal veins (number of patients=7), that the structure was profoundly changed. Thickening of the vessel wall, marked increase in extracellular material, disruption of the cytoarchitecture consisting in fragmentation of smooth muscle cells bundles, which showed a general disorganization, were the proeminent changes observed in the varicose veins. Moreover, the smooth muscle cells of the varicose tissue exhibited some alterations, namely hypertrophy (as indicated by a significant increase in mean cell dimensions) *(Table I)* and signs of an increased protein synthesis (exuberant nuclei and rough endoplasmic reticula).

After incubation with 0.1µmol/l of 3H-noradrenaline, the autoradiographs of the varicose and the normal vein again showed a very different picture

Table I. – Human saphenous veins

	Control	n	Varicose	n
Smooth muscle cell diameter	4.57 ± 1.90	945	6.98 ± 2.51*	783
Volumetric density of smooth muscle	38.0 ± 7.9	9	25.3 ± 3.7*	8

*Statistically different from control $p<0.001$

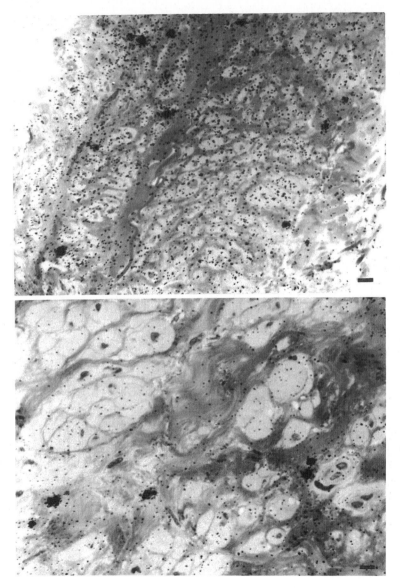

Figure 1. – Light microscope autoradiographies of human saphenous vein strips incubated with ^{3}H-noradrenaline (0.1µmol/l) for 30 min. In the control vein (A) clusters of silver grains indicative of adrenergic varicosities are seen throughout the whole media. Smooth muscle cells exhibit quite a high density of silver grains. In the varicose vein (B) nerve varicosities are less abundant, smooth muscle cells are larger and have a much lower density of silver grains and collagen is more abundant. Bars=10µm.

(Fig. 1). Not only was the density of silver grain clusters corresponding to adrenergic varicosities strikingly reduced in the varicose vein, in comparison to control (normal) vein tissue, but the labelling of extraneuronal cellular elements markedly reduced.

Finally, varicose veins differed from their normal counterparts in their endogenous noradrenaline content. In fact, whereas normal veins had a content of $0.32 \pm 0.02 \mu g/g$, the varicose veins had less than half that content, namely $0.14 \pm 0.01 \mu g/g$ (n=7 for each, P<0.01).

Canine veins

The morphological study of the veins revealed a number of differences between the vessels obtained from young or from old animals, mature dogs often occupying an intermediate position. Briefly, the volumetric density of smooth muscle cells decreased with age, from 45 % in young animals to 20 % in the old dogs. The diameter of smooth muscle cells increased from young to mature animals and decreased again in old animals, in which it attained values similar to those observed in young animals.

Noradrenaline content had a similar behaviour to that of volumetric density of smooth muscle. In fact, the vessels of young animals showed a maximal content (of about $4.5 \mu g/g$), whereas veins obtained from old animals had a content of only $1.9 \mu g/g$. Again, mature animals occupied an intermediate position ($2.8 \mu g/g$). All these results were obtained in groups of 4 to 6 animals.

The effects of sympathetic denervation (which resulted in a decrease of noradrenaline content of 93-97 %) on the morphology of veins were indistinguishable in the animals belonging to different age groups. The denervated veins consistently exhibited an increase in wall thickness, due both to hypertrophy of the cells and augmented extracellular material. Moreover, smooth muscle cells had a large, indented nucleus, augmented euchromatin and an increased rough endoplasmic reticulum ; fibroblasts were increased both in number and in dimensions and mast cells (absent from the normal canine saphenous vein) made their appearance.

Discussion

It is our intention to briefly discuss three points : the differences observed between the normal and the varicose human vein, the age-related changes of the canine vein and the comparison between the changes due to denervation of the canine vein and the alterations which varicose disease brings to the human venous tissue.

Although the main morphologic changes observed in varicose veins are well known and our results are in good agreement with those reported by Rose [1], there are some points which appear to merit special attention. In fact, apart from the classical changes due to increase in extracellular material and disorganization of smooth muscle cell bundles, we found a significant hypertrophy of smooth muscle cells and morphological signs of an increased protein synthesis. Moreover, the varicose vein showed a reduced density of adrenergic varicosities, as demonstrated by the lessened accumulation of ^{3}H-labelled noradrenaline, confirmed by the decreased content of endogenous noradrenaline. Thus, the varicose vein behaves like a partially denervated vein.

Since varicose disease is age-related, it appeared of interest to study the changes in structure of the canine vein attributable to ageing. Our study proves that age-related changes are evident in the canine saphenous vein : decrease of volumetric density of smooth muscle cells and progressive decrease in endogenous noradrenaline content, indicating lessened sympathetic innervation. The impact of surgical sympathetic denervation on the structure of the vein was consistent in all age groups : hypertrophy of smooth muscle cells, increased production of extracellular material and hypertrophic and hyperplastic changes of fibroblasts, accompanied by the appearance of mast-cells (absent from control veins).

Taken together, our observations allow to draw some analogies between the human varicose vein, the canine vein of " old " dogs and the denervated canine vein. *Table II* gives an overview of the similarities (and dissimilarities) of these vessels. Perusal of *Table II* clearly shows that the human varicose vein shows a number of similarities to both the saphenous vein of old animals and the denervated vein. Thus, the suggestion advanced earlier [5] that the denervated saphenous vein of the dog appears to be a model for the human varicose vein finds additional support in the present results. The only important differences lies in the fact that the human varicose vein is characterized by a decreased volumetric density of smooth muscle cells, since this does not happen in the denervated vein. However, the veins of old animals have a decreased volumetric density of smooth muscle cells, and it is tempting to assume that these veins after denervation probably represent the closest experimental model for the human varicose vein.

In conclusion, the human varicose vein behaves like a partially denervated vessel and many of its structural and biochemical peculiarities appear to be linked to the reduced sympathetic supply of the vein. The denervated canine vein represents an interesting model for the study of the human varicose vein.

Table II. – Similarities and dissimilarities of human and canine veins.

	Varicose human vein	Canine "old" vein	Denervated canine vein
Dimensions of smooth muscle cell (SMC)	+	0	+
Volumetric density of SMC	-	-	0
Endogenous noradrenaline content	-	-	--
Labelling of adrenergic terminals by ^{3}H-noradrenaline	-	?	--
Extracellular material	+	+	+
Metabolism of noradenaline	-	?	--

Signs : - reduced; -- markedly reduced; + increased; ? - not studied; 0 - without change

References

1. Rose S. (1986) The aetiology of varicose veins. *In : Phebology' 85,* D. Negus and G. Jantet (eds). John Libbey and Co Ldt, 1986; pp 6-9.
2. Branco D, Albino-Teixeira A, Azevedo I, *et al.* Structural and functional alterations caused at the extraneuronal level by sympathetic denervation of blood vessels. Naunyn-Schmiedeberg's Arch Pharmacol 1984; 326 : 302-312
3. Azevedo I, Osswald W. Trophic role of the sympathetic innervation. J Pharmacol (Paris), 1986; 17 Suppl 11 : 30-43.
4. Dimitriadou V, Aubineau P, Taxi J, *et al.* Ultrastuctural changes in the cerebral artery wall induced by long-term sympathetic denervation. Blood Vessels 1988; 25 : 122-143.
5. Branco D, Osswald W. The influence of *Ruscus* extract on the uptake and metabolism of noradrenaline in the normal and varicose human saphenous vein. Phlebology 1988 ; 3 Suppl 1 : 33-39.
6. Azevedo I, Castro-Tavares J, Garrett J. Ultrastructural changes in blood vessels of perinephritic hypertensive dogs. Blood Vessels 1981; 18 : 110-119.
7. Sarmento A, Soares-da-Silva P, Albino-Teixeira A, *et al.* Effects of denervation induced by 6-hydroxydopamine on cell nucleus activity of arterial and cardiac cells of the dog. J Auton Pharmac 1987; 7 : 119-126.
8. Teixeira A Albino, Azevedo I, Branco D, *et al.* Sympathetic enervation caused by long-term noradrenaline infusions; prevention by desipramine and superoxide dismutase. Br J Pharmacol 1989; 97 : 95-102.
9. Azevedo I, Osshaldf W. Uptake, distribution and metabolism of isoprenaline in the dog saphenous vein. Naunyn-Schmiedeberg's Arch Pharmacol 1976; 295 : 141-147.

Return circulation and Norepinephrine : an update. Ed. P.M. Vanhoutte. John Libbey Eurotext, Paris © 1991, pp. 139-150.

14

Structure of healthy and varicose veins

**H. Bouissou, M. Julian, M.-Th. Pieraggi, E. Maurel,
J.-C. Thiers, L. Louge**

*Service d'Anatomie Pathologique, CHU Rangueil, Chemin du Vallon,
31054 Toulouse Cedex, France*

This paper describes the morphology of the long saphenous vein, most affected by varicosis, according to age and condition. The microscopical and ultrastructural characteristics of the healthy and of the varicose vein, both young and aged, have been reviewed [1-5]. These earlier reviews are completed here by immunofluorescence study of type I and III collagens and biochemical study by extraction and measurement of total collagens I, III, IV, V and VI.

Morphological study

A structural review of the saphenous vein was carried out through the study of 31 macroscopically normal saphenous veins obtained at autopsy from normal subjects (25-92 yr) and 41 varicose saphenous veins, three obtained from autopsies and 38 during surgery (26 women aged 24-65 yr, 12 men aged 25-92 yr). For the former, samples were taken 4 cm from the saphenofemoral junction and 10 cm from the tibial crest; for the latter, samples were taken from dilated varicose segments and from macroscopically normal segments.

139

Young healthy veins (Figures 1, 2)

The young and healthy vein can be observed up to the age of 50 or 60 years. Its structure is practically identical in the tibial and in the femoral portion, the only difference being the more constant thickness of the media in the leg. In the media, beneath a thin intima, three musculo-fibrous layers can be distinguished : the internal layer is thin, and contains smooth muscle cells (SMC) perpendicular to the lumen, lying longitudinally and separated by loose collagen with some elastic fibers; the middle layer, which is the thickest of the three, is made up of numerous bundles of SMC, circular and concentric, separated by a small amount of collagen and by short elastic fibers; the external layer is a transitional zone where the limits are not clearly defined between the media and the adventitia. It contains islets of longitudinal SMC, clearly separated by thick fibrous tissue with distinct, continuous,

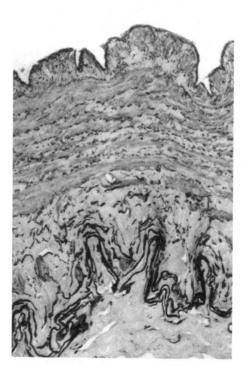

Figure 1. – Healthy saphenous vein. The very thin intima is separated from the media by a slender, continuous elastic layer. Short, slender elastic fibers are regularly distributed throughout the thickness of the media between the muscular bundles. In the outer zone, several concentric layers of thick elastic lamellae are visible (Verhoeff's haematoxylin x 10).

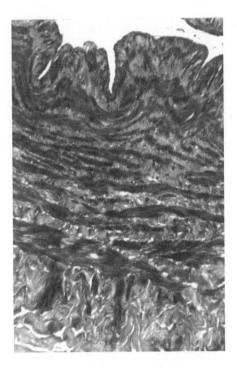

Figure 2. – Healthy saphenous vein. The three muscular layers of the venous wall can be clearly seen : a thin longitudinal inner wall, a wide middle layer with concentric muscular bundles. In the outer zone, a considerable amount of collagenous tissue is present between the longitudinal islets of muscular cells (Masson's trichrome stain x 10).

concentric and parallel elastic laminae. The fibrous adventitia merges into the connective tissue surrounding the vein.

Electron microscopy *(Figure 3)* confirmed these data and mainly revealed the contractile phenotype of the SMC.

Immunofluorescence demonstrated the predominance of type I collagen over type III in the three tunicas of the vein.

Aged healthy veins (Figures 4, 5)

The age-linked changes in the wall appear between 50 and 60 years, later than those of the corresponding artery, the tibial artery. They are less stereo-

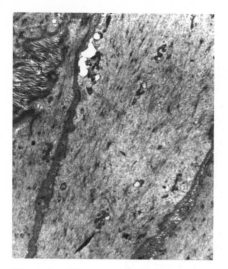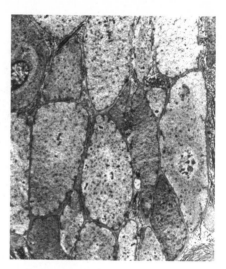

Figure 3. – Electron microscopy of a young healthy vein. *Left* The media consists of contractile SMC, seen in longitudinal section and separated by spare collagen (Uranyl acetate – lead citrate stain x 5 000). *Right* Young healthy vein, external media. " Cell nests " viewed in cross-section and surrounded by membrane-like material (Uranyl acetate – lead citrate stain x 4 000).

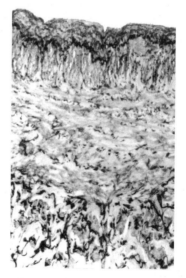

Figure 4. – Aged saphenous vein. The thickening of the intima is clearly visible. The internal elastic lamina is split. The elastic fibers of the media are reduced in number and irregularly arranged. The outer elastic layer is disrupted. The elastic fibers are thin, fragmented, dystrophic and randomly oriented (Verhoeff's haematoxylin x 10).

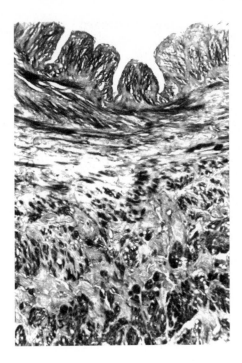

Figure 5. – Aged saphenous vein. Fibrous thickening of the intima. Fibrosis of the media. The internal muscular layer is not affected. The circular muscular bundles are broken up and disappearing. Increase of the externa longitudinal islets (Masson's trichrome stain x 10).

typed and vary in intensity from one segment to another and from one subject to another. They lead to :

— Sub-intimal fibrous thickening.

— Fibrosis of the three musculo-fibrous layers of the media, which however remain distinct. This fibrosis is atrophic, since the measurements of eight young healthy veins (mean age 27 ± 2 yr) and eight aged healthy veins (mean age 79 ± 3 yr) showed a distinctly significant decrease ($p<0.001$) in the thickness of the age wall. Measurements made from the intima to the external medial layer inclusive were on average $918\pm11\mu$ in the young subjects and $777\pm12\mu$ in the aged subjects.

— An overall decrease in elastic tissue, accompanied by dystrophic changes in the fibers and the various elastic lamellas, in particular in the outer layer of the media.

— Atrophy of the middle muscular wall and hyperplasia of the SMC in the cell nests of the outer layer of the media.

Electron microscopy *(Figure 6)* showed the SMC are mainly of the contractile type. Some take on a secretory phenotype especially in the external cell nests. They are then surrounded by a band of membrane-like material (probably type IV and VI collagens). In the media, the intercellular connective tissue shows some abnormalities in diameter (flower collagen).

Immunofluorescence showed that type I collagen was predominant throughout the wall, though type III was also present.

Young and aged varicose veins (Figures 7, 8)

We have already indicated [2] that there are no definite morphological differences between the dilated and non-dilated segments of the varicose vein and that the structural and organizational anomalies of the varicose wall differ from those of the aged vein. The varicose vein has three characteristics, regardless of age and sex :

— disorganization of the entire wall by dense and continuous fibrosis,

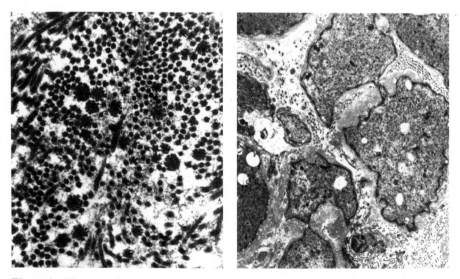

Figure 6. – Electron microscopy of an aged saphenous vein. *Left* In the media, the collagen fibers are very irregular and show flower fibrils (Uranyl acetate – lead citrate stain x 15 000). *Right* External media. "Cell nests" with SMC viewed in cross-section, surrounded by thick membrane-like material (Uranyl acetate – lead citrate stain x 5 000).

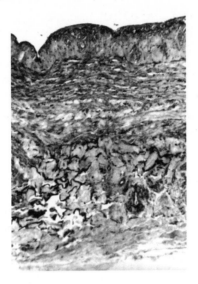

Figure 7. – Varicose saphenous vein. Throughout the media, decrease, dystrophy and disorganization of the elastic network (Verhoeff's haematoxylin x 10).

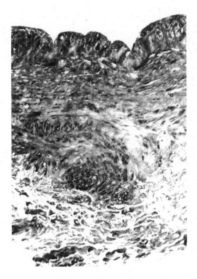

Figure 8. – Varicose saphenous vein. The wall is disrupted by dense fibrosis. The muscular layers show anarchic distribution with irregular bundles randomly aligned and thickening of the fibrous tissue between the bundles (Masson's trichrome stain x 10).

145

— decrease in the elastic network which becomes dystrophic,

— breakdown of the structure of the muscular layers (especially the middle layer) with scarcer of hyperplastic SMC bundles.

Ultramicroscopy *(Figure 9)* showed abundant collagen. It separates the SMC and its fibers show many anomalies. At certain points the SMC, of secretory phenotype, are surrounded by a thick band of membrane-like material.

Immunofluorescence showed that type I collagen was predominant, with a small quantity of type III collagen.

Origin of fibrosis : a problem

By light microscopy, in the young healthy vein, some stellate cells can be seen in the framework of connective tissue between the muscle bundles. These cells are extremely rare in the aged vein. Bloom and Don Fawcet [9] observed the presence of scare fibroblasts in the venous wall but did not indicate the age of the veins. In spite of our many ultramicroscopic examinations, we have never been able to affirm the presence of these cells. The venous wall however contains SMC of secretory phenotype. Can we assume that SMC alone are responsible by their secretory activity for the collagen framework observed in all human veins ? It should be borne in mind that in the artery fibroblasts are absent and that the interstitium is entirely secreted by SMC though it does not have the same importance as in the vein.

In the varicose vein, we have never observed with certainty the presence of fibroblasts. On the other hand, active dedifferentiated cells with a well-developed ergastoplasm are seen. They may be considered to be of muscular origin as vestiges of basal membrane and/or a highly indented nucleus and/or rare intracytoplasmic dense areas remain. In addition, the cells are often disorientated and surrounded by collagen fibers, whereas in the normal vein, whether young or aged, they are aligned either lengthwise or in a circular fashion according to the three constitutional muscular layers to which they belong.

Biochemical study

In order to remove the collagens soluble in acid and in neutral solutions, the fresh tissue of each homogenized vein was treated first with a neutral and

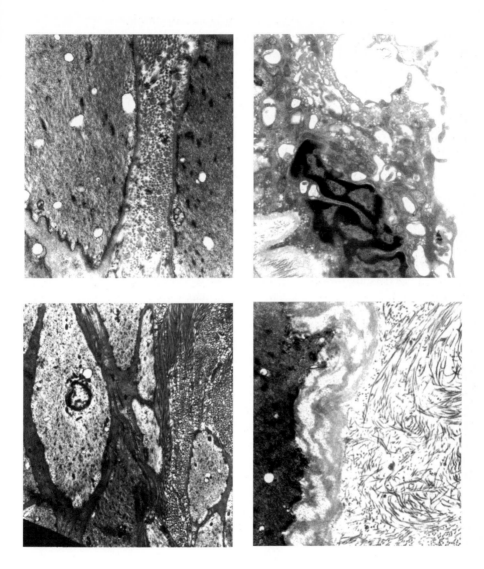

Figure 9. – Electron microscopy of a varicose vein. *Top left :* Media : contractile SMC are separated by collagen showing numerous irregularities of diameter (Uranyl acetate – lead citrate stain x 10 000). *Top right :* Outer media : highly dedifferentiated cell (secretory SMC) surrounded by abundant collagen (Uranyl acetate – lead citrate stain x 7 000). *Bottom left :* Media : cell nests with SMC surrounded by thick membrane-like material; abundant collagen (Uranyl acetate – lead citrate stain x 5 000). *Bottom right :* Detail of the membrane-like material surrounding some SMC. Layered, wavy appearance of this material in contact with collagen (Uranyl acetate – lead citrate stain x 10 000).

then with an acid buffer. The residue was subjected to pepsin digestion. Collagen was precipitated by a concentration of 0.7 M NaCl. The precipitate contained type I and III collagens and the supernatant type IV, V and VI collagens. In each fraction, collagen was quantified by hydroxyproline measurement (method of Bergman an Loxley) [6]. Typing was carried out by polyacrylamide gel electrophoresis (interrupted method of Sykes *et al.*) [7].

In previous publications [2, 8], we analysed (all ages being pooled) 15 healthy veins (mean age 54±5 yr) and 14 varicose veins (mean age 46±4 yr) simultaneously on apparently normal and on dilated segments. Varicose veins showed an increase (p<0.001) in total collagens, types I and III. The quantities of the other collagens (IV, V and VI) were analysed together because of the small quantities of each which were extracted. The value obtained was also significantly higher (p<0.001) than in normal veins.

In the present study, we analysed eight young healthy veins (21-33 yr) and ten aged healthy veins (65-92 yr), ten young varicose veins (25-38 yr) and eight aged varicose veins (59-78 yr). The results are given in *Tables I* and *II*. In the normal vein *(Table I),* the quantity of type I and III collagens was increased (p<0.001) in aged subjects as compared with young subjects. The minor collagens (types IV, V and VI) did not vary. In the varicose vein *(Table I),* no significant differences appeared with age. *Table II* shows that in the young subject, type I collagen content was identical in the normal and in the varicose vein; that type III collagen and the minor collagens decreased (p<0.001) in the young varicose vein; and that in aged varicose veins, type I and III collagens increased (p<0.01) as did the minor collagens (p<0.02).

Table I. – Collagen types evaluation with aging in normal (NV) and varicose vein (VV).

	Young	p	Aging
NV	(8)		(10)
Type I	648	<0.001	344
Type III	114	< 0.001	60
Others	152	NS	144
(IV, V, VI)			
VV	(10)		(8)
Type I	505	NS	522
Type III	84	NS	84
Others	267	NS	232

Table II. – Collagen types of normal and varicose saphenous veins in young (Y) and old (O) patients.

	Normal vein	p	Varicose vein
Y	(8)		(10)
Type I	648	NS	505
Type III	114	<0.01	84
Others IV, V, VI	152	< 0.01	267
O	(10)		(8)
Type I	344	< 0.01	522
Type III	60	< 0.01	84
Others	144	< 0.02	232

Conclusions

Comparison of the aged and the healthy vein demonstrates the existence of an ageing process in the vein leading to atrophic sclerosis of the wall.

The malformative morphological characteristics of the varicose vein appear at varying ages according to their intensity and are certainly related to the way of life of the subject, in particular profession, obesity, pregnancies, phlebitis, etc. The predominance of dense fibrous tissue, disorganization of the wall with diminished, dystrophic elastic tissue and the presence of disrupted, hyperplastic or dystrophic muscular layers (especially the middle layer), are the morphological characteristics which differentiate the varicose vein from a normal aged vein. The varicose vein is thus a dysplastic vein.

Even at an early age, the wall of a varicose vein has a lower collagen content than that of a healthy subject of the same age, but a higher level than that of a normal aged subject. This collagen content does not vary with age. These biochemical results confirm that the varicose vein is of dysplastic origin and not merely acquired.

References

1. Cabanne F, Bonenfant JL. Anatomie Pathologique. Paris : Maloine, 1986.

2. Bouissou H, Julian M, Pieraggi MT, *et al.* Les aspects tissulaires de la veine saphène interne normale, vieillie et variqueuse. Artères et Veines 1988; 7 : 431-435.

3. Bouissou H, Julian M, Pieraggi MT, *et al.* Vein morphology. Phlebology 1988; 3 : 1-11.

4. Bouissou H, Julian M; Pieraggi MT, *et al.* Les varices essentielles de la saphène interne. Bull Acad Natl Med 1988; 172 : 529-534.

5. Orcel L. *In : Anatomie pathologique vasculaire,* p 170h-170k, 1978. Paris : Flammarion Médecine-Sciences, Orcel L and Chomette G, Eds.

6. Bergman I, Loxley R. Two improved and simplified methods for the spectrophotometric determination of hydroxyproline. Anal Chem 1963; 35 : 1961-1967.

7. Sykes B, Puddle B, Francis M, *et al.* The estimation of two collagens from human dermis by interrupted gel electrophoresis. Biochem Biophys Res Commun 1976; 72 : 1472-1480.

8. Maurel E, Azéma C, Deloly J, *et al.* Collagen of the normal and the varicose human saphenous vein : a biochemical study. Clin Chim Acta 1989 (under review).

9. Bloom W, Don Fawcet W. A text book of histology. Philadelphia, W.B. Saunders Company 1962.

Return circulation and Norepinephrine : an update. Ed. P.M. Vanhoutte. John Libbey Eurotext, Paris © 1991, pp. 151-156.

15

Biochemical investigations on the action of *Ruscus* extract and trimethylhespiridinchalcon (TMHC)

V. Seydewitz, D. Berg, P. Welbers, J. Staubesand

Albert-Ludwige Universität, Albertstrasse 17, 7800 Freiburg, Germany

Introduction

The development of a varicose vein is associated with typical changes in the vessel wall. In comparison with the situation in the healthy vein there is an increase in glycosaminoglycans and in the activity of several lysosomal enzymes, which play a part in the catabolism of glycosaminoglycans [1-3]. At the same time, characteristic degenerative changes in the varicose vein manifest themselves ultrastructurally in the collagen [4] and elastic fibers, and this contributes significantly to loss of elasticity of the vein wall, and of other mechanical properties which characterize the normal vessel [5-7].

We therefore decided, because of this interaction between the proteoglycans, collagen and elastin, to investigate the possibility that *Ruscus* extract and THMC, substances which have a protective effect on veins, might exert an influence on the activity of β-N-acetylglucosaminidase (β-NAG) – a key enzyme in proteoglycan catabolism – and also on the activity of elastase and acid and alkaline phosphatase in the varicose great saphenous vein. Whereas the first three enzymes are predominantly localised in the lysosomes of

151

smooth muscle cells as acid hydrolases, alkaline phosphatase is largely membrane-bound, and plays a part in the calcification of blood-vessel walls [8]. Our earlier biochemical investigations on venous transplants enabled us to establish that there is a marked difference in the activity of enzymes in the proximal and distal segments on a vein. In the present study we have therefore estimated the activity of these enzymes in the two regions of these veins from groups of treated and untreated patients.

Material and methods

We examined women (36 patients) with varicosities of stage IV (HACH) of the main trunk of the great saphenous vein and with stage I or stage II chronic venous insufficiency (CVI) : indications for surgical stripping. The duration of history of the conditions was about 15 years. These patients were on average 43 years old, weighed 66 kg and were 165 cm in height. Each of the women had also had on average two pregnancies.

Patients were excluded from the investigation on the grounds of acute thrombosis, varicose ulcer, post-thrombotic syndrome, severe renal or hepatic insufficiency, angina pectoris, marked hypotonia, obliterative disease of the peripheral arteries, treatment with diuretics, pregnancy or heavy smoking (>30 cigarettes/day).

The design of the investigation consisted in a randomised double-blind experiment that was carried out for 4 weeks before the stripping operation. Seventeen patients received 3 capsules daily containing 150 mg *Ruscus* (standardized to contain 3.75 mg ruscogenin) and 150 mg TMHC, and 19 patients were given a placebo (lactose).

The degree of pain experienced in the knee – as reported by the patient – was recorded on a five-stage scale both before and after surgery.

During the operation, two segments of vein 2 cm in length were removed and kept for estimation of the enzyme activity ; one segment being taken from the upper end of the great saphenous vein just below its termination ("crosse"), and one from the region of the ankle. These specimens were kept in the deep-freeze at −20° C until required for assay.

Assay of the enzyme activity was carried out spectrophotometrically, with appropriate modifications : β-NAG [9]; Elastase [10]; acid and alcolin phosphatase, [11]. The specific enzyme activity is given in mU/mg protein. Protein was estimated with bovine serum albumin as the standard [12]. Statistical analysis was carried out, unless otherwise stated, with the Mann-Whitney U-test and a significance level of $p < 0.05$ recorded.

Results

In the placebo group, the enzyme activity values were always higher in the distal segment than in the proximal region of the vein. The higher values in comparison with the "crosse" region were statistically significant for the activity of β-NAG and alkaline phosphatase *(Figure 1)*. On the other hand, the protein content (proximal, 5.16 mg/ml; distal, 3.94 mg/ml), which was used as the reference value for calculating the specific activity of the enzymes, was significantly lower in the distal segment.

A 4-week treatment with *Ruscus* and TMHC brought about an increase of enzyme activity in the proximal segment, accompanied by a slight fall in the distal segment. A significant difference between the two segments could no longer be demonstrated *(Figure 2)*. If the differences in enzyme activity or protein content between the two segments ("crosse" minus ankle-region) of all patients are compared, the treated group shows significantly lower values

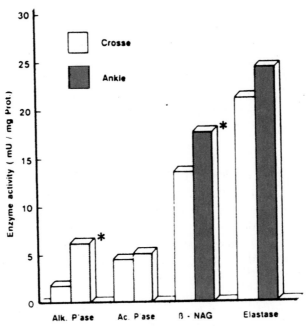

Figure 1. – Mean values of the specific enzyme activity in the proximal ("crosse") and distal (ankle) regions of the greath saphenous vein in placebo group. *=significantly higher enzyme activity (β-NAG p<0.019; Alk. P'ase p<0.0342) in the ankle region measured by Mann-Whitney test.

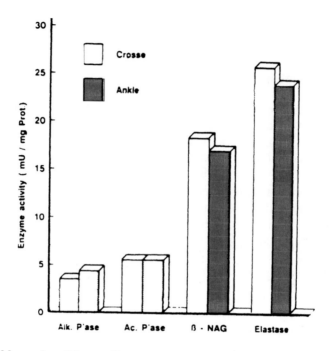

Figure 2. – Mean value of the specific enzyme activity in the proximal ("crosse") and distal (ankle) regions of the great saphenous vein in treated group. Result of treatment : increase in enzyme activity in the proximal region, so that the difference between the two venous segments is no longer significant.

Table I. – Differences in enzyme activity (Crosse minus Ankle). Great saphenous vein : varicosity stage IV (Hach)

Enzyme	$\overline{x}$	Placebo SE (n=19)	$\overline{x}$	Drug SE (n=17)
β-NAG	−4.14	1.22*	1.35	0.82
Alk. P'ase	−4.41	1.95*	−0.91	2.65
Ac. P'ase	−0.64	0.60	0.02	0.34
Elastase	−3.19	1.84	1.86	2.27
Protein (mg/ml)	1.22	0.43*	−0.33	0.18

* p<0,05 Mann - Whitney U-Test.

Table II. – Assessment of pain

Treatment	improved*	not improved**	total cases
Drug	9	7	16
Placebo	2	13	15
Total	11	20	31

* pain less severe after 4 weeks treatment
** pain the same or worse than before treatment
Fischer test p<0.023

for β-NAG, alkaline phosphatase and protein, whereas the difference for elastase is not significant and acid phosphatase remains unchanged *(Table I)*.

The questioning of patients about the severity of their pain before and after treatment revealed a distinctly higher incidence of subjective improvement in the drug group *(Table II)*.

Discussion

The target group for this combination of *Ruscus* and TMHC includes patients with CVI of stage I and II. Since we needed specimens of veins for the biochemical investigations, the study was carried out on patients with clinical indications for the stripping operation. In spite of the severity of the varicosity in such patients, the significance of the action of this drug combination on the protein content and the activity of β-NAG and alkaline phosphatase could be established.

Whereas in the placebo group, constantly higher values of the specific enzyme activity were recorded for the haemodynamically more severely loaded ankle region, a marked increase of specific enzyme activity was found in the proximal segment in the drug group after treatment. The reduction in protein content, which we used as a reference for the specific enzyme activity, can account for this, since the two are related inversely one to another.

In other words, the more heavily loaded distal segment is less able to respond to medication than the relatively unburdened proximal segment. Since, however, in the untreated group, the proximal segment is not protected by the therapy, its protein content remains in comparison with the other group relatively high, and it is because of this that the specific enzyme activity is apparently less than in the treated group.

We interpret the reduction of the extracted protein as indicating increased stabilization of the cell membranes within the wall of the varicose vein. It therefore seems likely that reduction of pain may indeed be the result of the medication.

References

1. Buddecke E. Chemie und Stoffwechsel des Venengewebes. Therapiewoche 1976 ; 26 : 5088-5099.

2. Laszt L. Zur Biochemie der Venenwand. *In* : Leu H.J. (Hg.) *Die Venenwand.* Huber, Bern-Stuttgart-Wien 1971.

3. Niebes P, Laszt L. Recherches sur l'activité des enzymes dans le métabolisme des mucopolysaccharides des veines saphènes humaines et bovines. Angiologica 1971 ; 8 : 7-16.

4. Zwillenberg LO, Laszt L, Zwillenberg H. Die Feinstruktur der Venenwand bei Varikose. Angiologica 1971 ; 8 : 318-346.

5. Staubesand J. Matrixvesikel und Mediadysplasie : Ein neues Konzept zur formalen Pathogenese der Varikose. Phlebol u Proktol. 1978 ; 7 : 109-140.

6. Staubesand J, Seydewitz V. Zur formalen Pathogenese der Varikose. *In :* Wuppermann T. (Hg) *Varizen, Ulcus cruris und Thrombose.* Springer, Berlin - Heidelberg - New York - Tokyo 1986.

7. Staubesand J, Seydewitz V. Morphologische Merkmale der varikösen Venenwand bei Stammvarikose. Schattauer, Stuttgart-New York 1989.

8. Seydewitz V, Staubesand J. Calciumbestimmungen, enzymbiochemische Untersuchungen an Saphenaven von Patienten mit Foronarsklerose oder Varikose. Z gesamte inn Med 1990 ; 45 : 100-103.

9. Barrett AJ, Heath MF. Lysosomal enzymes. *In :* Dingle J.T. (Ed.) *Lysosomaes, a laboratory handbook.* North-Holland, Amsterdam - New York-Oxford 1977.

10. Starkey P. Elastase and cathepsin G ; the serine proteinase of human neutrophil leucocytes and spleen *In :* Dinge J.T., Barrett A.J. (Eds.) *Proteinases in mammalian cells and tissues.* Elsevier, North-Holland Biomedical Press 1977.

11. Walter K, Schütt C. Saure und alkalische Phosphatase im Serum. *In :* Bergmeyer H.U. (Hg.) *Methoden der enzymatischen Analyse.* Verlag Chemie, Weinheim 1974.

12. Lowry OA, Rosenbrough NJ, Farr A, *et al.* Protein measurement with folin phenol reagent. J Biol Chem 1951 ; 193 : 265-275.

Return circulation and Norepinephrine : an update. Ed. P.M. Vanhoutte. John Libbey Eurotext, Paris © 1991, pp. 157-162.

16

Influence of *Ruscus* extract* and methylhesperidine chalcone on the fibrinolytic activity of the vein wall

S. Haas, G. Lill, A. Stiller, K. Geißdörfer, G. Blümel

Institut für Experimentelle Chirurgie, Klinikum rechts der Isar, Technische Universität, München, Germany
Chirurgische Abteilung, St. Eduardus-Hospital, Köln, Germany

Introduction

The treatment of varicose veins make up a large portion of the day-to-day work of the general practitioner and the dermatologist. They are not only a cosmetic problem for the patient but, in addition to their pathophysiological significance for the development of chronic venous insufficiency (CVI), they constitute a risk factor for the development of thrombosis. With respect to pathogenesis, the augmented frequency of thrombosis in varicose veins is probably connected with a reduced level of tissue plasminogen activator (t-PA) in the wall of the varicose vein. The use of drugs which normalize this state of deficiency is thus of great clinical relevance.

Ruscus extract* has been used routinely for many years in the treatment of venous disease of various etiology. However, the effect of this drug on tissue

---

* Phlebodril®

fibrinolysis has not been investigated to date. Therefore, the present study was designed to determine whether or not this drug can stimulate the production of t-PA in the venous wall.

Materials and methods

Patients

The investigation was designed as a placebo-controlled double-blind study with randomized administration of verum or placebo capsules. Before beginning the study the approval of the institutional ethic committee was obtained. The following inclusion criteria were defined : age 30 to 65 years, CVI state I or II caused by a primary varicosis and valvular incompetence of the great saphenous vein in male or female patients. The exclusion criteria were : post-thrombotic syndrome, CVI state III, interfering concomittant medication in the two weeks proceeding surgery (aspirin, drugs for venous conditions or for improvement of blood-flow, oral contraceptives, systemic cortisone), phlebography in the two weeks proceeding surgery, insulin dependent diabetes mellitus or other manifest metabolic disease. After verification of the inclusion and exclusion criteria the patients were informed about the nature and scope of the study. Informed consent was obtained.

One capsule of the active drug form contained 150 mg extr. rhiz. *Ruscus aculeatus* (standardized to 3,72 mg ruscogenin) and 150 mg methylhesperidine chalcone (MHC). One capsule of the placebo form contained the corresponding amount of lactose. The treatment covered a period of 14 days. One capsule was administered three times daily. The last capsule was taken on the evening before surgery.

Collection and processing of vein segments

Intra-operatively a 1 cm segment was excised as atraumatically as possible from the great saphenous vein and a further 1 cm segment from a varicose vein. Particular attention was taken to avoid mechanical damage to the vascular segments by forceps and strippers. Immediately after removal the tissue samples were shock-frozen and stored at -20°C until further work-up.

The fibrinolytic activity of the vascular segments was examined by means of fibrinolysis autography according to Todd [1]. In this technique a cryocut section of venous wall is incubated for various lengths of time at 37°C on a fibrin film containing plasminogen. Depending on the amount and release of the plasminogen activator contained in the tissue the plasminogen in the underlying fibrin film is activated to plasmin leading to dissolution of the fibrin film. After fixing and staining of the slide the areas of fibrino-lysis appear as pale unstained areas within the dark-coloured fibrin layer [2].

The fibrinolytic activity of intima and adventitia were determined separately after an incubation period of 30,60 and 90 min.

According to Pandolfi three degrees of lysis can be distinguished [3]. In degree I lysis the fibrin layer is only slightly lighter in colour. In degree II lysis the areas of fibrinolysis are larger, the dissolution of the fibrin layer reaches as far as the slide. In degree III lysis there is a massive dissolution of the fibrin layer. The areas of fibrinolysis merge and tissue particles float away so that the tissue structures are scarcely identifiable in places.

The statistical analysis was performed using the Mann-Whitney-U-Test.

Results

The two patient groups did not differ significantly according to age, sex, height or body weight *(Table I)*.

After an incubation time of 60 and 90 min the fibrinolytic activity of the intima of the great saphenous vein was significantly increased in the active drug group (p<0.01) *(Figure 1)*. The adventitia layer of the great saphenous vein showed a significant increase after an incubation time of 60 min

Table I. – Characteristics of patients

	Verum x (SD)	Placebo x (SD)
Number of males	1	4
Number of females	9	6
Age (years)	61.4 (7.3)	48.1 (10.2)
Weight (kg)	62.6 (8.0)	73.0 (11.8)
Height (cm)	165.0 (7.0)	172.0 (8.0)
History of disease (years)	23.0 (6.8)	19.5 (7.2)

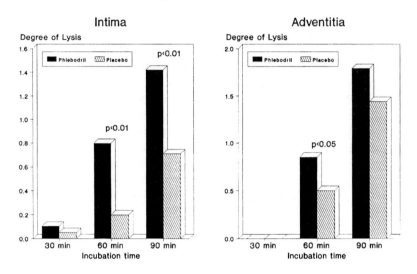

Figure 1. – Fibrinolytic activity during the fibrinolysis autography test. The vein segments were excised from patients with chronic venous insufficiency state I or II and valvular insufficiency of the great saphenous vein.

($p<0.05$). After incubation for 90 minutes we were only able to identify a trend in this direction but statistical confirmation was not possible as the variance of data was too great.

In segments form peripheral varicose veins no significant increase in t-PA activity was found at any incubation time in the patient group treated with *Ruscus* extract.

Discussion

Within the venous circulation clots are composed mainly of fibrin-rich material. Under physiological conditions they are prevented by the release of t-PA from the vascular endothelium. In the varicose vein the fibrinolytic acti-vity is markedly reduced [4]. Thus in patients with varicose veins throm-boses are nine times higher than in a healthy population [5].

Apart from numerous risk factors for the development of thrombosis, such as advanced age, marked obesity, severe varicosis, excessive nicotine consump-tion and hormone treatment, there are several additional circumstances which can favor the development of thrombosis such as immobilization of the lower extremity of insufficient use of the ankle and muscle pump. A combination of risk factors and unfavorable circumstances potentiates the risk of thrombotic complications in patients with varicosis. In order to re-duce the risk of thrombotic processes it would be useful to take a venous drug which stimulates the release of endogenous t-PA.

In the present study we were able to show for the first time that the combina-tion of *Ruscus* extract and MHC stimulates the production of t-PA in the ve-nous wall. Despite the small number of patients, the finding in the great sa-phenous vein appear quite clear, due samples to the homogeneity of the tissue specimens. These veins segments were all removed from the same lo-cation, i.e. as close as possible to the junction with the femoral vein. The morphology of the vein is thus uniform in all patients.

The results in the segments from peripheral varicose veins show conside-rable variation. Here the various degrees of severity, different durations of illness, the different sites of the varicose veins and thus the differences in morphological structure may be of major importance. Nevertheless, the re-sults of this study provide a foundation for further investigations in which the fibrinolysis-increasing action of *Ruscus* extract should be experimentally and clinically corroborated.

The enhancement of fibrinolytic activity may contribute to a faster healing of venous ulcers [6]. At least the time period for healing up of ulcers and there-fore the stay in hospital was shortened significantly by a *Ruscus* extract treatment [7].

References

1. Todd AS. The histological localisation of fibrinolytic activator. J Path Bact 1964 ; 78 : 281-283.
2. Nilsson JM, Isacson S. Effect of treatment with combined phenformin and ethyloestrenol on the coagulation and fibrinolytic system. J Clin Pathol 1972; 25 : 638-639.
3. Pandolfi M. Histochemical and assay of plasminogen activator (s). Rev europ Etud Chir et Biol 1972; 17 : 254-260.

4. Büttner D. Schmidt FC. Die fibrinolytische Aktivität der Venenwand. Vasa 1972; 1 : 24-28.

5. Widmer LK, Stähelin HB, Nissen C, *et al.* Venen, Arterien-Krankheiten, koronare Herzkrankheit bei Beruistätigen. Hans Huber, Bern Stuttgart, Wien 1981.

6. Burnand KG, Browse MD. Use of fibrinolytic enhancement in the treatment and prevention of recurrent venous ulceration. Practical cardiology 1983; 9(11) : 229-237.

7. Leyh F. Therapie des Ulcus cruris venosum mit Mäusedornextrakt und Trimethlyhesperidinchalkon : Ergebnisse einer Doppelblindstudie. Therapiewoche 1988 ; 38 (33) : 2325-2331.

Return circulation and Norepinephrine : an update. Ed. P.M. Vanhoutte. John Libbey Eurotext, Paris © 1991, pp. 163-169.

17

Effect of *Ruscus* extract* in chronic venous insufficiency stage I, II and III

H. Kiesewetter, P. Scheffler, F. Jung, J. Schwab,
J. Blume*, M. Gerhards****

Department of Clinical Haemostasiology and Transfusion Medicine,
** *Medical and Out-Patient Hospital, Internal Medicine II,*
University of the Saarland, D-6650 Homburg-Saar, Germany
*** *Center for Cardiovascular Diseases, Alexianergraben 9,*
D-5100 Aachen, Germany

Introduction

Venous diseases are a problem of social medicine [2, 6]. The basic therapy of chronic venous insufficiency consists of physical therapy as for example swimming, isometric exercises, pedal ergometric exercises with elevated legs and walking on soft underground, cold affusions and compression therapy, either elastic wraps (only a limited time) or compression stockings made to measure in case of edemas or marked varicosis, respectively. Blood is pumped more easily toward the heart and the venous hydrostatic pressure is reduced by these measures. The additional administration of a venous therapeutic agent in order to contract the veins and to reduce the permeabi-

---

*Phlébodril® (Lipha Arzneimittel Gmb H)

lity of vein walls is discussed. All measures mentioned and drug therapy reduce the edema and thus the subjective feeling of tension and heaviness. Perception disorder, pain and calf cramps are symptoms which can be eliminated only on a long term basis [1, 3]. In the study presented here the efficacy of *Ruscus* extract was tested.

Patients

The subjects (n = 30) were selected at random from a group of patients with chronic venous insufficiency (CVI). Mean body height of the patients with CVI I (11 women, 4 men) was 169.5±6.4 cm, mean body weight 71.9±12.2 kg, and mean age 50.6±12.0 years. The average number of births was 1.9. 40 % worked in a standing position. Two patients were adipose, 1 had diabetes mellitus, 3 were smoking, 3 were hypertensive and 1 presented another concomitant disease. Mean body height in the group with CVI II, III (12 women, 3 men) was 170.0±5.5 cm, mean body weight 66.5±6.9 kg, and mean age 55.1±14.5 years. The average number of births was 2.3. Sixty per cent worked in a standing position. Three presented adiposity, 2 diabetes mellitus, 6 were smoking, 3 hypertensive and 5 had other concomitant diseases.

Group I (CVI I) consisted of 5 patients with primary varicosis (stage I and II) and 10 with chronic venous insufficiency stage I. Group II (CVI II, III) included the patients with chronic venous insufficiency stage II and III. Both groups consisted of 15 patients.

Methods

During the last years prior to the study all patients were treated insufficiently. Therefore, they had to undergo physical measures over the first eight weeks of treatment. Then, all patients were additionally treated with *Ruscus* extract over a period of five months. The most important clinical parameters measured in this study were : circumference of the legs, subjective symptoms of pain and venous capacity. Besides, rheological and haemostasiological parameters as well as some protein concentrations were measured. During the first five weeks the drug therapy consisted of 3x2 *Ruscus* extract capsules, then 2x2 capsules a day *(Figure 1)*.

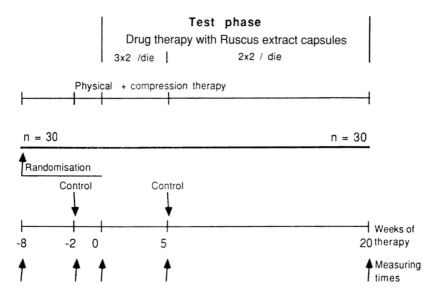

Figure 1. – Illustration of study schedule

The subjective symptoms were determined by means of analogous scales (severity of complaints ranging between 0-100). A "venous index" was formed with an average of all venous symptoms. To study normal distribution the Kolmogoroff-Smirnow test was used. In multiple samples the test for time series of angiological and rheological parameters was used as global test (Friedmann test).

Results

Patients with CVI

The circumference of the lower legs decreased by about 0.5 cm (not statistically significant) by the physical measures (measuring times –8 to 0) *(Figure 2)*. During the last two weeks of the prephase (measuring times –2 to 0) they did not change. A significant decrease by 1.2 cm could only be

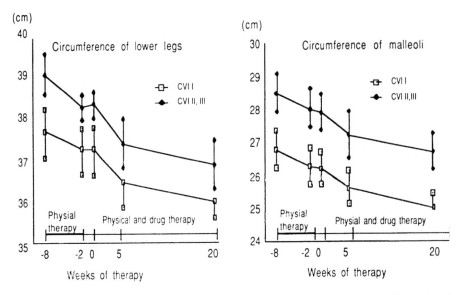

Figure 2. – Decrease in the circumferences of malleoli and lower legs during the 28 weeks of the study. After eight weeks of physical therapy alone the patients received additional drug therapy (mean value ± standard error of the mean).

achieved by the additional drug therapy (p≤0.01) (measuring times 0 to 20); a significant decrease was already found after five weeks (p≤0.01) (measuring time 5).

Similar changes were observed concerning the malleolar circumferences (not significant). The decrease was about 0.5 cm after physical therapy and another 1.2 cm after additional therapy with active substance (p≤0.01) *(Figure 2)*.

The changes after the eight weeks of prephase (measuring times – 8 to 0) were not significant. The reductions in venous capacity were 0.7 ml/100 ml-tissue after five weeks of *Ruscus* extract treatment and 0.9 ml/100 ml-tissue after five months of therapy *(Figure 3)*.

The rheological values for the patients with CVI I were within the normal range. The rheological parameters did not change significantly with treatment.

Patients with CVI, II, III

In this group, a main decrease (p≤0.01) in the circumferences of the lower legs and malleoli was already achieved by the compression therapy in com-

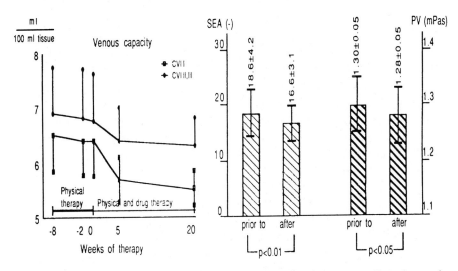

Figure 3. – Venous capacity of both groups during the treatment phase as well as plasma viscosity (PV) and erythrocyte aggregation (SEA) in patients with CVI, II, III prior to application and after five months (mean value ± standard error of the mean).

bination with physical therapy (measuring times –8 to 0). A further significant reduction in the circumferences of the legs could be attained by the following administration of active substance (measuring times 0 to 20). The total decrease in malleolar circumferences was 1.9 and 2.15 in the lower legs *(Figure 2)*. During the course of drug therapy (measuring times 0 to 20) the venous capacity decreased significantly ($p \leq 0.01$) by about 10 % to values of about 6.2 ml/100 ml-tissue. Plasma viscosity and erythrocyte aggregation were reduced by 1.5 % and 10.8 % respectively after five months of therapy *(Figure 3)*.

The complaints were reduced markedly especially during the first five weeks of medication ("venous index" changed from 40 to 14). The following treatment brought about an additional reduction (from 14 to 9). In all, there was a significant reduction by about 78 % ($p \leq 0.001$).

Discussion

Prior to the treatment phase both groups presented a decrease in the circumferences of the lower legs (significant in patients with CVI, II, III) and a reduction of subjective complaints which was achieved by physical measures. Then, there was a stagnation during the last two weeks of this phase. During the following treatment phase of five weeks with additional application of active substance the circumferences of the lower legs, subjective complaints, and venous capacities continue to reduce.

The initial situation of the patients with CVI, II, III is worse than that of the patients with CVI I both concerning the circumferences of the lower legs and malleoli. This was to be expected due to the more marked lesions of the first-mentioned group; surprising, however, is the similar improvement in both groups. In any case, the decreases are within similar ranges and thus the curves of both groups are almost parallel.

The decrease in venous capacity corresponds well with the experimental results found by Rudofsky [4]. In spite of the relatively long duration of drug therapy the values are hardly reduced after five weeks treatment.

The positive effect of physical measures turns clearly out on measuring the circumferences of the lower legs and malleoli. This effect is supported by the additional drug therapy. The significant decrease in the circumferences of the patients with CVI, II, III seems to be especially important. This is revealed by the changes in the " venous index " which is determined by means of a scale on which patients report the subjective severity of their complaints. This is most pronounced if the initial circumferences are already relatively elevated. Thus, it can be explained that this index decreases by more than 80 % in group with CVI, II, III and, in spite of elevated initial values, is even significantly below the index of the CVI I-group after the treatment phase.

All results described so far indicate improved haemodynamics achieved by the test therapy. Moreover, the additionally performed investigation of rheological parameters demonstrate that pharmaceutical therapy improves the fluidity of blood.

These results found *ex vivo* seem to be remarkable as they confirm the results of previous *in vivo* studies. In both studies it was found that the improvement in fluidity is mainly due to a decrease in erythrocyte aggregation. Although the absolute changes are small it must be considered that blood fluidity is considerably worse in the affected venous areas with disturbed outflow than in the blood of the cubital vein. Thus, rheological improvements in the lower extremities could be more marked and partly be the reason for the reduction of the complaints.

References

1. Felix W, Schmidt G, Nieberle J. Protektive Wirkung von Trimethylhesperidinchalkon und *Ruscus aculeatus* genenüber dem Etracrynsäureödem am Hinterlauf der narkotisierten Katze. Phlebol u Proktol 1983; 12 : 209-218.
2. Fischer H. Socio-epidemiological study on distribution of venous disorders among a residential population. Inter Angio 1984; 3 : 89-94.
3. Marcelon G, Vanhoutte PM. Mechanism of action of *Ruscus* extract. Inter Angio 1984; 3 : 74-76.
4. Rudofsky G. Die Wirkung einer oralen Gabe von Dihydroergotamin auf das kaudale Venensystem. Herz-Kreislauf 1985; 2 : 90-93.
5. Volger E ; Öller J, Pfafferott C. Hydrostatischer Venendruck und lokale hämorhoelogisch Störung beim postthrombotischen Syndrom. 6. Kongreß der Dtsch. Ges. für Klin. Hämorheologie, Essen, Oktober 1987.
6. Widmer LK, *et al.* Venenerkrankungen bei 1800 Berufstätigen. Basler Studie II. Schweiz med Wschr 1967; 97 : 107.

Return circulation and Norepinephrine : an update. Ed. P.M. Vanhoutte. John Libbey Eurotext, Paris © 1991, pp. 171-179.

18

Action of *Ruscus* extract* cream in the treatment of acute sport injuries

D. Böhmer

Sportmedizinisches Institut, Frankfurt am Main e.v.,
Otto Fleck Scheise 10, 6000 Frankfurt 71

With the growth of leisure-time sporting activities, there has also been an increase in the number of sport injuries. 20 % of all accidents are already accounted for by sport injuries. Fortunately, very few of them require surgical treatment. By far the majority of cases are contusions and *sprains*. These are associated with hematomas, hemarthrosis, soft tissue injuries without external wounds, and pain with restriction of movement. The initial treatments to avoid the formation of effusions and edemas are immobilization, cooling, compression, and elevation. In addition, topical administration of anti-inflammatory drugs accelerating absorption is advisable, firstly to counteract any inflammatory reaction and secondly to rapidly eliminate the hematoma and edema, so as to restore mobility and eliminate pain. The edema-reducing effect of *Ruscus* extract as the therapeutically active constituent of *Ruscus* extract cream has been demonstrated in extensive animal experiments [1, 2] and in clinical studies on volunteers [3, 4] and patients with venous diseases [5, 6]. *Ruscus* extract also has an anti-inflammatory action [7]. The prophylactic administration of *Ruscus* extract significantly reduced postoperative swelling [8, 9] and accelerated the absorption of hematomas [10]. *In vitro* studies [7] and volunteer studies [11,12] have demonstrated that there was

---

* Phlebodril®

adequate active substance penetration of skin into soft tissue, blood vessels and lymph vessels. The anti-oedematous, lymphokinetic and anti-inflammatory properties of melilot extract [13, 14], the second therapeutically active substance is *Ruscus* extract, potentiate the effects of the melilot.

On the basis of its known pharmacological effects it can therefore be assumed that *Ruscus* extract cream accelerates the absorption of hematomas and edemas in sport injuries, particularly minor sports injuries, and thus promotes restoration of mobility. The substance was therefore tested in a randomized double-blind study in patients with sprains and contusions of the knees and ankles.

Patients and methods

Sixty patients were enrolled in the study. Twelve patients did not meet the inclusion and exclusion criteria. These patients were therefore included only in the evaluation of tolerability. The remaining 48 patients, aged between 16 and 53 (median 29 years) had sprain or contusions of the lower leg or the foot. Twenty six patients were treated with *Ruscus* extract cream and 22 received a placebo of identical appearance. Both groups of patients were comparable in terms of sex distribution and severity of injury. Severe contusions or sprains with suspected torn ligaments constituted an exclusion criterion. There were slight differences between the groups in the location of the injuries.

Patients with open wounds as a result of the sport injury were not included in the study. In addition, it was not permitted to take any analgesic or anti-inflammatory in addition to the test substance during the 14-day test phase. Physical measures were also not to be used.

The treatment given was 3x4 g cream daily, applied to a large area of the affected limbs. Vigorous massage was to be avoided. 100 g *Ruscus* extract cream contains 1.6 g *Ruscus* extract and 1.6 g melilot extract.

For an objective assessment of the outcome of treatment, the force that could be applied without pain, the circumference, and the skin temperature on the injured and uninjured sides were determined. Pain at rest, pain on movement, and pain on pressure were assessed on a four-point scale.

The target criteria were checked between the 3rd and 5th days of treatment and at the end of treatment after 14 days.

In the statistical evaluation the difference in muscle strength, circumference, and skin temperature between the injured and uninjured sides was checked with analysis of variance with repeated measurements. The significance level for the study was set at α=0.05.The p values for the statistical test were adjusted according to the number of tests performed after Bonferroni.

The pain symptoms were evaluated on a descriptive basis. Fisher's exact test was used to describe the differences between the groups.

Results

On enrolment in the study there were no major differences between the two groups of patients in terms of the maximally available muscle strength in the injured extremity (active medication group 24.3 kg, placebo 27.3 kg), circumference of the affected area (active medication 35.1 cm, placebo 35.4 cm), or the skin temperature (active medication 30.3°C, placebo 30.4°C). In both test groups the injury-related symptoms improved during the 14-day treatment period, but under active medication the improvement was more rapid.

The difference in the available muscle strength was reduced by 73 % under active medication. At the end of treatment the difference between the injured and the healthy extremity was only 8.9 kg. Taking into account the difference between the force exerted by the playing leg and the other leg, this difference can be regarded as virtually normal. Under placebo treatment the difference in muscle strength at the end of treatment was still more than double (18.5 kg, decrease 32 %) *(Figure 1)*.

The difference in circumference between the injured and uninjured sides decreased to the same extent in the active medication group, from on average 2.4 to 0.9 cm (by 63 %), whereas under the placebo the difference in circumference only decreased from 2.2 to 1.6 cm (27 %) *(Figure 2)*.

The skin temperature was on average 1.7°C higher than in the contralateral area in both patient groups at the start of the treatment. After treatment for 14 days the difference in temperature under active medication had decreased by 1.3°C (77 %). In the placebo group a decrease of only 35 % (0.6°C) was measured *(Figure 3)*.

The differences between the two groups in all three target criteria were highly significant (p<0.001).

The pain associated with the trauma was reduced more rapidly in the active medication group than in the placebo group. The effect of *Ruscus* extract cream in promoting healing was particularly pronounced in the assessment of pain at rest and on movement during the first few days of the treatment

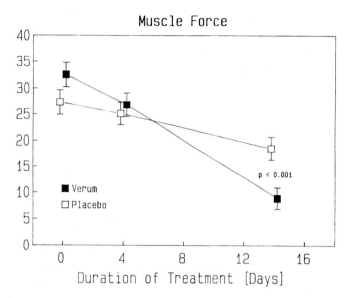

Figure 1. – Change of muscle force; difference between traumatized and healthy side : mean (x) and standard error (SE) of mean.

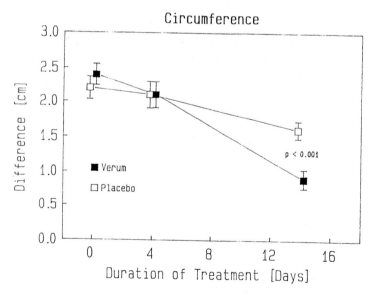

Figure 2. – Decrease of circumference; difference between traumatized and healthy side : mean (x) and standard error (SE) of mean.

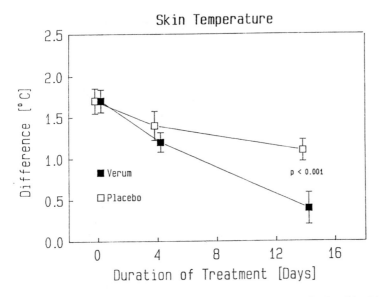

Figure 3. – Reduction of skin temperature; difference between traumatized and healthy side : mean (x) and standard error (SE) of mean.

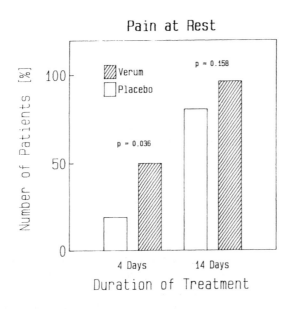

Figure 4. – Improvement of pain at rest.

175

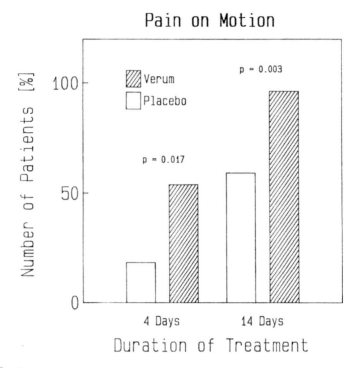

Figure 5. – Reduction of pain symptomatics on movement.

(Figures 4 and 5) (p<0.05). There was, however, also a tendency for pain on pressure to be reduced *(Figure 6)*.

The tolerability of the cream was assessed by all patients as good to very good; no adverse drug effects occurred.

Discussion

The tissue reaction after a contused injury showed the five classic signs of inflammation : redness, pain, swelling, elevated temperature, and restricted function. The above signs are due to a vascular reaction leading to hyperemia and increased release of mediators, amines and kinins released by various blood constituents (macrophages, monocytes, mast cells, etc.). These

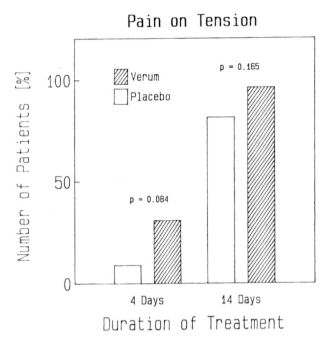

Figure 6. – Improvement of pain symptomatics on tension.

trigger and maintain the inflammation reactions in the tissue. Although this induces healing, residual reactions are common, and prolong the healing time.

In animal experiments [13] and in model studies in volunteers [7], melilot and *Ruscus* extract have been found to exert an anti-inflammatory action. The lowering of raised body temperature as a sign of a reduction in the inflammation reaction may be attributable to these anti-inflammatory properties of the active substances in the cream. Animal studies have also demonstrated that wound healing is accelerated by melilot extract [13].

The accelerated reduction in swelling can be attributed to two action mechanisms. In the first place, *Ruscus* and melilot extracts have a capillary-sealing action. As a result, escape of fluid into tissue is reduced. Secondly, the α-adrenergic action of *Ruscus* extract increases lymph vessel motricity [15]. As a result of macrophage stimulation by the benzopyrones and flavonoids in melilot extract [16], breakdown of proteins and hematomas in the intestinal area is accelerated.

The anti-edematous and antiexudative action of the active medication cream has a decisive effect on painful symptoms, particularly in the first few days

177

of the treatment. Strength tests provide objective proof that exercise tolerance recovers sooner as a result of the regression of swelling. This is a significant time advantage, particularly for working patients.

Conclusion

The antiexudative, lymphokinetic, and anti-inflammatory action of *Ruscus* extract cream significantly reduces the pain due to contused sport injuries. *Ruscus* extract cream should therefore be used as early as practicable, to produce a remission or at least an improvement.

References

1. Felix W, Nieberle J, Schmidt G. Protektive Wirkung von Trimethylhesperidinchalkon und *Ruscus aculeatus* gegenüber dem Etacrynsäureödem am Hinterlauf der narkotisierten Katze. Phlebol u Proktol 1983; 12 : 209-218.

2. Hönig I, Felix W. Effect on the permeability of the isolated ear vein of the pig : a comparison between flavonoids and saponins. *In : Phlebologie'89,* Davy A., Stemmer R. (eds), pp 680-682 John Libbey, Eurotext Ltd. 1989.

3. Rudofsky G, Hirche H. Phlethysmographische Untersuchungen eines Venentherapeutikums bei wärmebedingten hämodynamische Veränderungen. Med Welt 1985 ; 36 : 145-149.

4. Rudofsky G. Venentonisierung und Kapillarabdichtung. Fortschr Med 107, 1989 ; 19 : 430-434.

5. Rieger H. Efficacy of a combination drug in patients with chronic venous insufficiency under orthostatic conditions. Phlebology 1988; 3 : Suppl. 1, 127-130.

6. Rudofsky G, Diehm C, Gruß J, *et al.* Wirksamkeit einer Kombination venoaktiver Substanzen bei Patienten mit chronisch venöser Insuffizienz im Stadium I. *In : Therapie der Venenerkrankungen,* Denck, H., van Dongen, R.-J.-A.-M. 73-92, TM-Verlag Hameln 1989.

7. Stüttgen G, Bauer E, Siebel H Th. Studies of pharmacokinetics and analytical pharmacology of cream containing and extract of *Ruscus aculeatus*. Inter Angio 1984; 3 : Suppl. 1, 91-94.

8. Trautwein R, Hallmeier B. Prophylaxe postoperativer Schwellungszustände nache Kniegelenksoperationen. Med Welt 1987; 38 : 1210-1213.

9. Elies S, Katzke D, Steinbach E. Zur Ôdemprophylaxe mit Steroid-Saponinen bei Septo-Rhinoplastiken. Extracta otorhinolaryngologica 1987; 9 (2) : 69-72.

10. Mauss H. Therapie der oberflächlichen Thrombophlebitis nach Verödung. Therapiewoche 1978; 37 (19) : 1792-1799.

11. Thebault JJ. Untersuchungen zur Wirkung eines Phlebotonikums. Forschr med 101 1983; 25 : 1206-1212.

12. Rudofsky G. Transkutane Venentonisierung und Kapillarabdichtung bei gesunden Proban-den. MMW 131 1989; 18 : 362-365.

13. Földi-Börczök E, Bedall FK, Rahlfs VW. Die antiphlogistische und ödemhemmende Wir-kung von Cumarin aus Melilotus officinalis. Arzneim-Forsch 1971; 21 (12) : 2025-2050.

14. Monographie Meliloti herba, Steinkleekraut, 18.02.1986.

15. Marcelon G, Pouget G, Tisné-Versailles. Effect of *Ruscus* on the adrenoceptors of the ca-nine lymphatic duct. Phlebology 1988; 3 : Suppl. 1, 109-112.

16. Casley-Smith JR, Casley-Smith Judith R. High protein oedemas and the benzopyrones. Lippincott Sydney; 1986.

Return circulation and Norepinephrine : an update. Ed. P.M. Vanhoutte. John Libbey Eurotext, Paris © 1991, pp. 181-196.

19

Sympathetic nervous control of tonus in large-bore arterial vessels, arterioles and veins, and of capillary pressure and fluid exchange in cat skeletal muscle (comparative effects evoked by *Ruscus aculeatus* extract)

S. Mellander, M. Maspers, U. Ekelund

*Department of Physiology and Biophysics, University of Lund,
Sölvegatan 19, S-223 62 Lund, Sweden*

Introduction

The various consecutive sections of the vascular bed from artery to vein subserve different vascular functions which by integrated interaction aim at the establishment of an optimal nutritional supply to the tissues under maintained overall cardiovascular homeostasis. This interaction, however, is complicated by the fact that the site of action of the different vascular control systems is not uniform along the vascular bed. For an understanding of this complex interplay there is a need of a reliable method which can provide simultaneous and quantitative information of the regulation of the different vascular functions in hemodynamically meaningful terms.

A method with this potential was recently developed in our laboratory which on a cat whole-organ muscle preparation for the first time permits continuous and simultaneous analyses of resistance responses in the whole vascular bed and in the following morphologically defined consecutive section : large-bore arterial resistance vessels (>25μm), arterioles (<25μm), and veins. In addition, it provides data for capillary pressure and fluid exchange. This method was here adopted for a description of the sympathetic nervous control with regard to : 1) the site and pattern of sympathetic action along the muscle vascular bed, 2) the magnitude of total and segmental resistance responses in the initial and in the steady-state phase of sympathetic activation, 3) the rate of resistance development in the different consecutive segments, and 4) the sympathetic control of capillary pressure and fluid exchange and the underlying changes of the ratio of pre- to postcapillary resistance. This study has been described at full length elsewhere [1].

A comparative study was also performed of the vascular effects in skeletal muscle of *Ruscus* extract, a drug considered to have a preferential constrictor action on the veins in the peripheral circulation [2].

Methods

Material and anaesthesia

Observations of sympathetic nervous effects were performed on 17 young adult cats (mean bwt 4.4 kg), and observations of effects of *Ruscus* extract were performed on 12 cats (mean bwt 5.0 kg). They were anesthetized intravenously with α-chloralose (50mg·kg^{-1} bwt). A tracheal cannula was inserted to facilitate spontaneous respiration.

Expiratory PCO_2 was monitored continuously and stayed within normal limits (4.5-5.5 kPa) during the experiment.

Skeletal muscle preparation and recordings

The lower leg muscles of the right hind limb were prepared as described in detail elsewhere [3, 4]. In brief, the muscle region was autoperfused in situ and regional arterial blood flow was recorded continuously with a differential pressure flowmeter. The muscle preparation was placed in a plethysmograph to permit volumetric recordings of capacitance responses and of net transcapillary fluid flux with a gravimetric volume recorder connected to a

Grass FT 10C transducer. Mean arterial inflow pressure (P_A) and venous outflow pressure (P_V) were recorded from T-tubes close to the popliteal artery and vein. P_V was set at a normal level which in the control state established an isovolumetric state (Starling fluid equilibrium) in the muscle preparation.

Measurements of capillary and arteriolar pressure were made from the lateral head of the gastrocnemius (LG) muscle according to a special microcannulation technique [3, 4] *(Figure 1)*. The studied LG muscle region is supplied by two segmental vascular circuits emanating from two side branches of the sural artery, of which the proximal circuit forms the main nutritional supply. Of special importance for the microvessel pressure measurements was the morphologically and functionally demonstrated existence of highly specific microvascular anastomotic connections between these two segmental vascular circuits. On the arterial side, these anastomoses consisted solely of arterioles of about 25μm (diameter) at normal vascular tone and on the venous side of capillaries and postcapillary venules of a size <10μm. For recordings of the microvascular pressures, fine catheters were inserted in the distal direction into the sural artery and vein, respectively, at a site between the described first and second side branches, and connected to pressure transducers. Distal pressure monitored under these circumstances from the sural artery ramifications was shown to represent hydrostatic pressure transmitted from the arteriolar anastomoses connecting the proximal and distal vascular circuits, thus representing pressure in ≈ 25μm wide arterioles ($P_{arteriole}$). Similarly, distal pressure monitored from the sural vein ramifications was shown to represent pressure transmitted from the numerous capillary/venular (<10μm) anastomoses, i.e. from a site very close to the main (venous capillary) fluid exchange vessels. This pressure, denoted $P_{C,V}$, thus should reflect average capillary pressure in the region which was verified[3] by observed close agreement with capillary pressure data obtained with other independent methods.

The four continuously recorded pressure signals (P_A, $P_{arteriole}$, $P_{C,V}$ and P_V) were fed into differential pressure transducers, thereby providing data for the total pressure drop across the whole vascular bed (P_A-P_V) as well as the segmental pressure drops from cognate artery to the arteriolar (≈25μm) level (P_A - $P_{arteriole}$), from arterioles to capillaries ($P_{arteriole}$ - $P_{C,V}$), and from capillaries to the popliteal vein ($P_{C,V}$ - P_V). These four differential pressure signals and the blood flow signal (Q), in turn, were fed into electronic analogue divider circuits (vascular resistance meters) to obtain continuous simultaneous recordings of total regional vascular resistance (R_T), proximal arterial resistance in vessels larger than about 25μm ($R_{a,prox}$), resistance in arterioles <25μm ($R_{a,micro}$), and venous resistance (R_V). Resistances were expressed in peripheral resistance units, PRU (mm Hg·ml^{-1}·min·100g tissue).

All parameters *(Figure 2)* were recorded on a 10-channel Grass Polygraph.

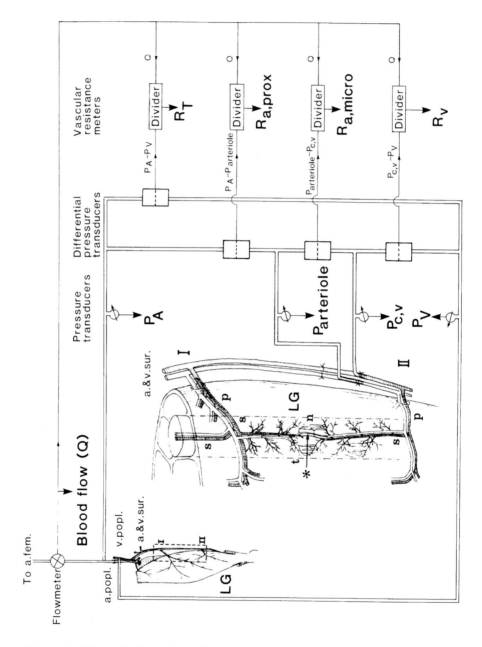

Figure 1. – Schematic illustration of the experimental approach used for segmental vascular resistance recordings in cat gastrocnemius muscle. Reproduced from reference 4 with permission.

Experimental protocols

The sympathetic vasoconstrictor nerves to the muscle region were excited by supramaximal stimuli (5 V, 5 ms) at rates from 1-16 Hz.

The presented data refer to sympathetic α-adrenergic constrictor effects since the stimulations were performed in the presence of atropine (1mg·kg^{-1} bwt, i.v.) and propranolol (1mg·kg^{-1} tissue, i.a.) for effective muscarinic and ß-adrenoceptor blockade, respectively. By a special approach [1], active and passive components in the segmental sympathetic constrictor responses could be distinguished and evaluated in quantitative terms.

Ruscus extract (Pierre Fabre Medicament) was infused close-arterially to the muscle region (7 cats ; n=24) in doses ranging from 0.1 to 6mg·min^{-1}·kg^{-1} tissue, at slow infusion rates (<0.2 ml·min^{-1}) to avoid infusion artifacts. *Ruscus* extract was also applied intravenously into the systemic circulation (5 cats, n=10) in doses ranging from 1-9mg·min^{-1}kg^{-1} bwt. Data are expressed as mean values $\pm$ SEM. Student's t-test was used for statistical evaluation, differences being considered significant at P-values <0.05.

Results

Segmental resistance responses to sympathetic nerve activation

Original recordings of the ten continuously measured circulatory variables are shown in *Figure 2* demonstrating the responses evoked by a short-term ($\approx$2 min) supramaximal stimulation of the sympathetic vasoconstrictor fibres to the skeletal muscle preparation at 8 Hz. The responses were obtained in the presence of regional ß-adrenoceptor and muscarinic blockade, thus aiming at investigating pure α-adrenergic effects. It can be seen that, nerve excitation caused an abrupt and marked decrease in blood flow (Q) to a steady state level reached within about 1 min. This was caused by a coordinated increase in total regional vascular resistance (RT) from the control value of 9.5 PRU to a steady state level of 57 PRU (6-fold increase). The sympathetic constrictor response was clearly confined to all three consecutive vascular segments. Note, however, that the arteriolar (<25μm) response (Ra,micro) developed much more quickly than the large-bore arterial resistance response ($R_{a,prox}$). Thus, from the control value of 3.2 PRU, $R_{a,micro}$ increased rapidly within 30 s to a peak value of 23.7 PRU (7.4-fold increase) followed by a partial relaxation, a so-called 'sympathetic escape phenomenon' down to a steady-state value of 20.2 PRU (6.3-fold increase). The $R_{a, prox}$ response

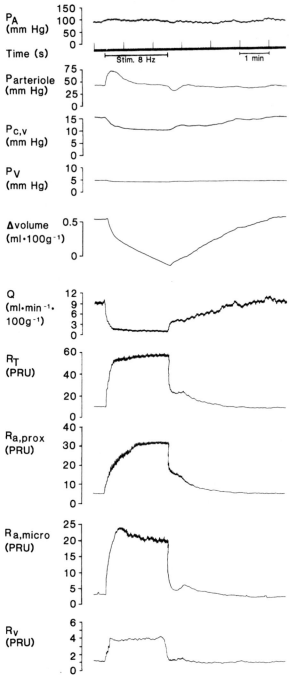

Figure 2. – Resistance responses in the whole vascular bed (R_T) and in large-bore (>25μm) arterial vessels ($R_{a,prox}$), arterioles (<25μm, $R_{a,micro}$) and veins (R_V) to sympathetic nerve stimulation at 8 Hz. Reproduced from reference 1 with permission.

was much more sluggish, rising gradually from a control value of 5.2 PRU to a steady-state value of 33 PRU in about 60s (6.3-fold increase). The sympathetic venous resistance response (RV), finally, was distinct and quite rapid in onset, reaching a steady-state value of 4.0 PRU within 15 s from the control value of 1.1 PRU (3.6-fold increase).

Although the adrenergic resistance response on the venous side (RV) was distinct, it was clearly smaller than that on the arterial side, hence leading to a neurogenic increase in the pre- to postcapillary resistance ratio. This latter adjustment has the important functional implication of controlling hydrostatic capillary pressure ($P_{C,V}$) which in this case decreased by 5.5 mm Hg from the control value of 15.7 mm Hg. This fall of P_C, in turn, caused a net transcapillary fluid absorption of $0.17 ml \cdot min^{-1} \cdot 100g^{-1}$ tissue, as derived from the late continuous decline of the tissue volume curve during steady-state sympathetic constriction.

Compiled data for peak (left bars) and steady-state (right bars) sympathetic constrictor responses are shown in *Figure 3*. The data are classed into three groups which can be considered to represent "slight" (1-2 Hz) "moderate" (4-6 Hz), and "strong" (8-16 Hz) sympathetic constrictor effects. It can be seen that sympathetic nerve excitation caused constriction in all three consecutive sections and that these responses were distinctly graded in relation to the excitation rate. Strong sympathetic stimulation caused in the steady state an average rise of RT from 15.3 to 120 PRU (7.8-fold increase). This overall effect was explained by a rise in $R_{a,prox}$ from 8.8 to 64 PRU (7.3-fold increase), a rise in $R_{a,micro}$ from 4.5 to 49 PRU (10.9-fold increase) and by a rise in R_V from 2.0 to 7 PRU (3.5-fold increase). This implied a considerable segmental redistribution of vascular resistance compared to control as shown by the numbers (% of R_T) within (or at) the bars in *Figure 3*, a greater fraction of resistance, in relative terms, being distributed to the $R_{a,micro}$ section. These resistance responses to sympathetic nerve activation were all found to be caused by active changes in vascular tonus, except for a minor (<10 %) passive component in the sympathetic venous resistance response [1].

The data in *Figure 4* illustrate the differences in the time-course of the sympathetic resistance development in large-bore arterial resistance vessels (O), arterioles (●) and veins (▲); in panel (a) expressed as time (s) from onset of stimulation to maximum constriction, and in panel (b) as rate of resistance development per unit time (PRU/s). Note from panel (b) the much greater rate of resistance development in the arterioles which, from a functional point of view, indicates a more efficient constrictor control of the arterioles than of the two other sections.

The data in *Figure 5* illustrate the extent of the sympathetically produced fall of capillary pressure ($P_{C,V}$) and the resulting rate of net transcapillary fluid absorption. In the pre-stimulatory control state (*Figure 5 : 0 Hz*), at

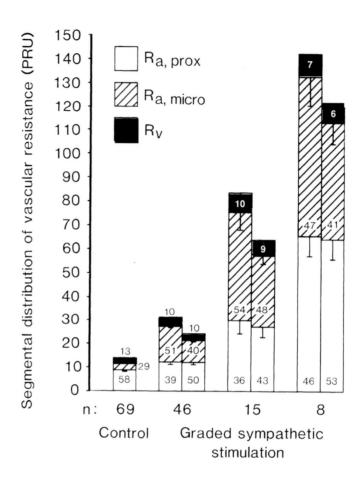

Figure 3. – Compiled data for segmental vascular resistance responses to "slight" (1-2 Hz), "moderate" (4-6 Hz) and "strong" (8-16 Hz) sympathetic stimulation (initial peak response, left bars; steady state response, right bars). Reproduced from reference 1 with permission.

R_T=17.2±0.3 PRU, $P_{C,V}$ for this material averaged 17.6±0.4 mm Hg and a Starling equilibrium (isovolumetric state) with zero net transcapillary fluid movement prevailed. Nerve stimulation caused an increasing capillary pressure drop with increasing rates of excitation and a consequent graded net transcapillary fluid absorption. The maximum fall of $P_{C,V}$, obtained at 16 Hz, averaged 6.9±0.5 mm Hg, and caused, in the steady state, net fluid absorption at a rate of 0.23±0.025ml·min^{-1}·100g^{-1} tissue. The capillary filtration coefficient (CFC) averaged 0.015±0.003ml·min^{-1}·100g^{-1}·mm Hg^{-1} in

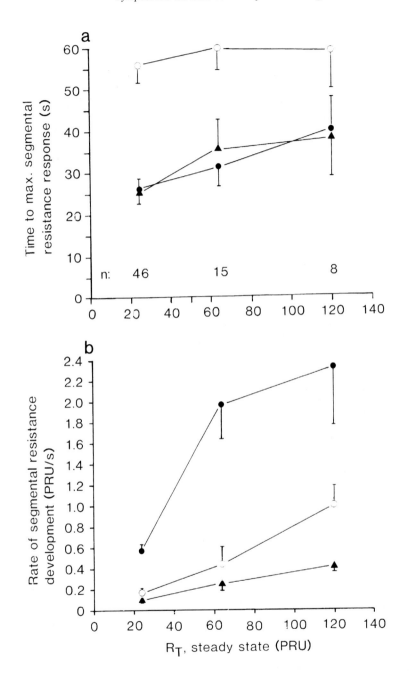

Figure 4. – Time course of the sympathetic resistance response in the $R_{a, prox}$ section (O), the $R_{a, micro}$ section (●) and veins (▲). Reproduced from reference 1 with permission.

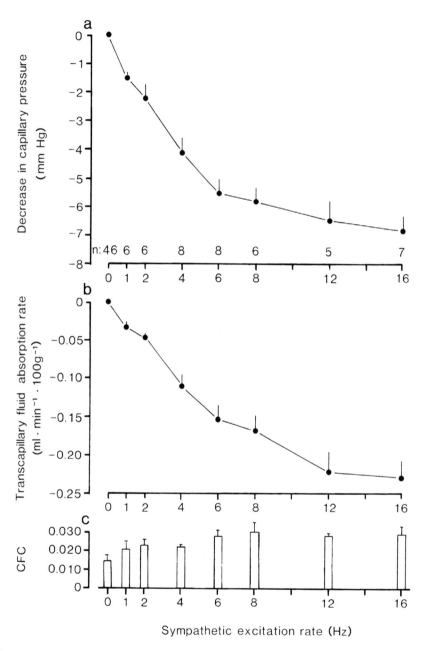

Figure 5. – Effects on capillary pressure, net transcapillary fluid absorption rate and capillary filtration coefficient (CFC) of sympathetic nerve stimulation at graded rates. Reproduced from reference 1 with permission.

the control period and tended to increase gradually with increasing rates of sympathetic stimulation *(Figure 5)*, indicating increased functional capillary surface area in the steady state of constrictor fibre influence.

Segmental resistance responses to the administration of *Ruscus* extract

Intra-arterial infusion

Original recordings of the effects of i.a. administration of *Ruscus* on overall regional vascular resistance (R_T), proximal arterial resistance in vessels >25µm ($R_{a,prox}$), arteriolar (<25µm) resistance ($R_{a,micro}$), venous resistance (R_V) and blood flow (Q) in cat skeletal muscle are shown in *Figure 6*. *Ruscus* infusion at a dose of $0.4mg \cdot min^{-1} \cdot kg^{-1}$ tissue elicited, within about 90 s a vasoconstrictor effect which raised R_T by about 30 % and influenced all three consecutive vascular segments, $R_{a,prox}$ increasing by 35 %, $R_{a,micro}$ by 23 % and R_V by 33 %. During continued infusion at this rate, the $R_{a,prox}$ and $R_{a,micro}$ responses tended to decline, whereas the R_V constrictor response was well maintained. The subsequent stepwise increase in the infusion rate which raised the dose of *Ruscus* to $0.8mg \cdot min^{-1} \cdot kg^{-1}$ elicited a marked initial blood flow increase and a decrease in R_T explained by marked dilator effects in all three vascular segments. This was followed by a remarkable oscillatory response pattern in all vascular segments during the remainder of the *Ruscus* infusion period, in which, over a period of about 50 s, resistance varied from very low values to such exceeding the control level. Cessation of the *Ruscus* infusion led to quick recovery of vascular tone in all sections.

Ruscus infusion at the dose of $3mg \cdot min^{-1} \cdot kg^{-1}$ tissue caused an initial constrictor response in all three vascular sections lasting for about 90 s, then suddenly followed by a very marked and now stable dilator response in all vascular segments, as summarized in *Figure 7* (n=4). During the initial constrictor response to *Ruscus*, R_T increased from an average value of 30.2±5.0 to 42.2±7.7 PRU, explained by a 39 % increase in $R_{a,prox}$, a 44 % increase in $R_{a,micro}$ and a 50 % increase in R_V. The subsequent sustained dilator response was associated with very marked inhibition of tone in all vascular sections.

This pattern of response in skeletal muscle with constrictor effects to low, and sustained dilator effects to high, concentrations of intra-arterially administered *Ruscus* was consistent in all experiments (n=24). Mention should be made that, in constrictor doses, *Ruscus* also caused a decline in capillary pressure by 1-2 mm Hg, whereas it rose transiently by up to 10 mm Hg during pronounced *Ruscus* dilatation, leading to transcapillary fluid absorption and filtration, respectively.

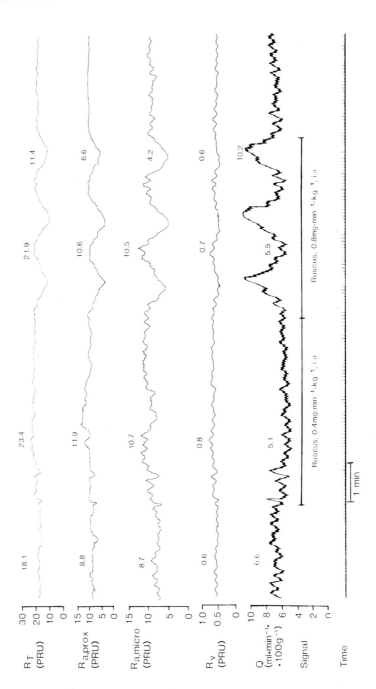

Figure 6. – Segmental vascular resistance responses in skeletal muscle to *Ruscus*.

Intravenous infusion

Ruscus was applied i.v. in doses ranging from 1-9mg·min^{-1}·kg^{-1} bwt. In the pre-infusion control period the following average values for vascular resistance in the muscle preparation prevailed : R_T 24.0±4.0, $R_{a,prox}$ 18.4±5.4, $R_{a,micro}$ 3.5±1.8 and R_V 2.1±0.4 PRU. The i.v. administration of *Ruscus* at a dose of 3mg·min^{-1}·kg^{-1} bwt (n=6) caused on the average an increase in R_T by 16 %, in $R_{a,prox}$ by 23 %, in $R_{a,micro}$ by 6 %, and in R_V by 6 %. The responses seemed to be dose-dependent; a high dose (9mg.min^{-1}·kg^{-1}) appeared to elicit an especially pronounced venoconstrictor response (43 % above control).

Discussion

The abundant sympathetic nerve supply to the vasculature of skeletal muscle shows a non-uniform distribution along the vascular bed from artery to vein as evidenced by electron microscopic and histochemical techniques [5]. The innervation density is greatest in the large-bore arterial vessels down to the level of small muscular arteries, quite pronounced also in the arterioles, more moderate in the terminal arterioles, and sparse or absent in precapillary sphincters, collecting venules, and muscular venules; it then increases again in the small and large veins.

Although such morphological evidence *per se* might indicate possibilities for a differentiated sympathetic control along the vascular bed, the ultimate net segmental constrictor responses to nerve excitation are determined by a number of additional factors, such as amount of norepinephrine release per unit smooth muscle mass [6], α-adrenoceptor density and sensitivity to the neurotransmitter [5], effects of Laplace's law [1], etc. The influence of these factors might very well differ between the various consecutive vascular segments. For an evaluation of the net outcome of such an interplay there is a need of functional studies of hemodynamically important variables during sympathetic activation.

The present methodology seems to provide a more comprehensive and detailed description than in the past of the sympathetic control of the vascular bed of skeletal muscle on the whole-organ level with regard to overall regional hemodynamics and effects on the arterial macro- and micro-circulation, capillary fluid exchange, and the venous circulation. The study showed that the extrinsic sympathetic nerves exert quite a generalized overall control of the large-bore arterial vessels, the arterioles and veins in skeletal muscle. This contrasts to the site of action of the local myogenic [4, 7] and metabolic [8] control systems, which, has been shown to be preferentially confined to the arteriolar section.

The described neural segmental vascular responses were all found to be active in nature, except for the sympathetic R_V response which included a minor passive component, comprising at most 10 % of the total response [1]. The demonstration of a pronounced active sympathetic regulation of the venous compartment in skeletal muscle is in agreement with previous detailed studies of the regulation of the capacitance function [9]. The present R_V analysis, however, is a much more selective and sensitive test of venous reactivity, since an arterial constrictor effect contributes to some extent to the capacitance response. The present results seem to distinctly refute the idea of Marshall [10] of a lack of active sympathetic control of the venous compartment in skeletal muscle. Her opinion was based on vital microscopic observations of diameter changes in selected venous microvessels, which might be a too insensitive method to reveal a moderate overall venous constriction.

Yet, the sympathetic control of the arterial side is more prominent than on the venous side, both in absolute and relative terms. This, among other things, has the functionally important consequence that nerve activation leads to an increased pre- to post-capillary resistance ratio which, in turn, forms the basis for the neural regulation of capillary pressure and fluid absorption, graded in relation to the nerve excitation rate *(Figure 5)*. If the present data *(Figure 5)* for the rate of net transcapillary fluid absorption at strong nerve excitation ($0.23 \text{ml} \cdot \text{min}^{-1} \cdot 100 \text{g}^{-1}$ tissue) were assumed to be representative for the whole muscle mass (1.3 kg) of the adult cat (3.5 kg), this would imply a plasma volume gain from the extravascular space of muscle of about 6 ml during a 2 min stimulation period. This corresponds to about 5 % of the animal's total normal plasma volume, which emphasizes the great potential for a prompt reflex sympathetic plasma volume control, for instance in bleeding.

The present comparative investigation of *Ruscus* extract effects revealed that the drug applied intra-arterially at low doses $\leq 0.5 \text{mg} \cdot \text{min}^{-1} \cdot \text{kg}^{-1}$) elicited moderate constrictions of large-bore arterial vessels, arterioles and veins in the muscle circulation. Similar effects were noted upon intravenous administration. These effects most likely can be attributed to a described $\alpha 1$-adrenergic component of the *Ruscus* response [2]. The cause of the pronounced generalized dilator reponse in skeletal muscle to close-arterial *Ruscus* administration at higher doses *(Figures 6, 7)* is not known but, speculatively, might be related to a *Ruscus* induced release of endothelium-derived relaxing factor (Miller *et al.*, this volume).

Ruscus is reported to be a therapeutically beneficial drug in various disorders with impaired venomotor function in humans [2]. Although the present fin-

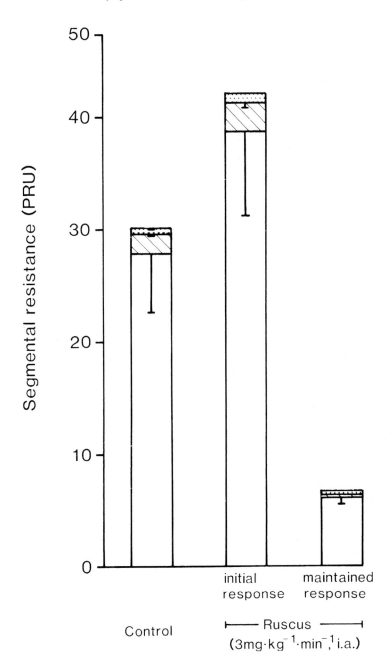

Figure 7. – Initial and maintained resistance response in the $R_{a,prox}$ ( ), $R_{a,micro}$ ( ) and R_V ( ) sections to a high dose (3mg·kg⁻¹·min⁻¹, i.a.) of *Ruscus*.

ding of a moderate venoconstrictor effect of the drug in the muscle circulation seems compatible with this concept, it appears form a quantitative point of view that the venous system of other vascular beds than skeletal muscle must be more important targets for *Ruscus* to fully explain a hemodynamically significant improvement of the venous return in states of disturbed venomotor function. The skin circulation could be of greater importance in this respect, since *Ruscus* has been shown to exert a very pronounced constrictor action on cutaneous veins *in vitro* [2].

Acknowledgement

The neural part of the study was supported by grant 2210 from the Swedish Medical Research Council.

References

1. Maspers M, Björnberg J, Grände PO, *et al.* Sympathetic α-adrenergic control of large-bore arterial vessels arterioles, and veins, and of capillary pressure and fluid exchange in whole-organ cat skeletal muscle. Acta Physiol Scand 1990; 138, In press.

2. Vanhoutte PM (ed). New advances in norepinephrine and veno lymphatic return. Phlebology 1988; 3 : suppl 1, 1-133. J. Libbey & Co Ltd, London.

3. Mellander S, Björnberg J, Maspers M, *et al.* Method for continuous recording of hydrostatic exchange vessel pressure in cat skeletal muscle. Acta Physiol Scand 1987; 129 : 325-335.

4. Björnberg J, Grände PO, Maspers M, *et al.* Site of autoregulatory reactions in the vascular bed of cat skeletal muscle as determined with a new technique for segmental vascular resistance recordings. Acta Physiol Scand 1988; 133 : 199-210.

5. Altura BM. Pharmacology of the microcirculation. *In : Microcirculation.* R.M. Effros, H. Schmid-Schönbein & J. Ditzel (eds). 1981, pp. 51-105. Academic Press, New York.

6. Mellander S, Johansson B. Control of resistance, exchange, and capacitance functions in the peripheral circulation. Pharm Rev 1968; 20 : 117-196.

7. Mellander S. Functional aspects of myogenic vascular control. J Hypertension 1989; 7 : suppl 4, S21-S30.

8. Björnberg J, Maspers M, Mellander S. Metabolic control of large-bore arterial resistance vessels, arterioles, and veins in cat skeletal muscle during exercise. Acta physiol Scand 1989; 135 : 83-94.

9. Mellander S. Comparative studies on the adrenergic neuro-humoral control of resistance and capacitance blood vessels in the cat. Acta Physiol Scand 1960; 50 : suppl 176, 1-86.

10. Marshall J. The influence of the sympathetic nervous system on individual vessels of the microcirculation of skeletal muscle of the rat. J Physiol 1982; 332 : 169-186.

Return circulation and Norepinephrine : an update. Ed. P.M. Vanhoutte. John Libbey Eurotext, Paris © 1991, pp. 197-205.

20

Pharmacological modulation of venular permeability with some antiinflammatory drugs

E. Svensjö

Department of Exploratory Pharmacology, Draco, Lund, Sweden

Introduction

Endothelial cells in culture respond to histamine and bradykinin stimulation with an immediate rise in intracellular concentration of Ca and inositolphosphates [1-4].

The functional response to receptor-mediated stimulation of endothelial cells *in vitro* could be demonstrated by measuring the passage of a macromolecular tracer (albumin) through widened cell junctions. In the same study it was also shown that histamine induced cytoskeletal changes in terms of a reduced F-actin content which is a sign of actin polymerisation and cellular contraction resulting in widened junctions or gaps [1].

These recent studies support the original proposal by Majno and Palade [5] that endothelial cells in postcapillary venules could contract on stimulation with serotonin and histamine. They demonstrated the escape of carbon particles, and by implication plasma leakage, from the vasculature at the level of postcapillary venules. The site of plasma leakage in the microvasculature has also been shown by combining intravital and electron microscopy of the same vascular bed [6]. Fluorescein labeled dextran (FITC-dextran,

MW=150,000) was given i.v. to hamsters and the cheek pouch microvasculature was observed by intravital microscopy. Extravasation of FITC-dextran (plasma leakage) was only observed in postcapillary venules after stimulation with bradykinin. The leaking venules were subjected to electron microscopy which could show electron dense precipitates of FITC-dextran in the vessel lumen, in the widened junctions (gaps) of postcapillary venules and in the interstitium [6].

The described technique of visualizing plasma leakage by intravital microscopy can show increased vascular permeability due to direct endothelial stimulation at the earliest 30 seconds after mediator application and will reach a maximum response at 3-5 min [7]. However, electrophysiological measurements of resistance of the endothelial cell lining in capillaries *in vivo* have shown that serotonin stimulation could reduce resistance within a second reaching a minimum within 10 seconds which is in analogy with the immediate response seen in cultured endothelial cells [8]. Measurements of nonstimulated arterioles and venules showed that there was a lower resistance on the venous side providing further evidence to why these vessels are more prone to leak [9]. Morphological studies have shown that a certain fraction, 25-30 %, of the intercellular junctions in postcapillary venules is open to a gap already under nonstimulated conditions [10].

The gathered view from *in vitro* and *in vivo* studies of endothelial cell functions supports the hypothesis that a physiological and pharmacological regulation of macromolecular permeability is exerted by the endothelial cells in the postcapillary venules [11-14]. This report will briefly describe the technique for vascular permeability studies in the cheek pouch preparation and give some results from studies on how the action of several inflammatory mediators could be modified by different pharmacological principles which probably act directly on the endothelial cells.

Material and methods

The use of the hamster cheek pouch for studies of macromolecular permeability has been described [7, 15, 16]. For microscopic observations the single layer cheek pouch preparation is performed essentially as described by Duling [17] with our modifications [16].

The hamster is anesthetized with pentobarbital and the cheek pouch is gently everted and mounted on the microscopic stage. The pouch is submerged in a pool and continuously superfused with a bicarbonate buffered saline solution

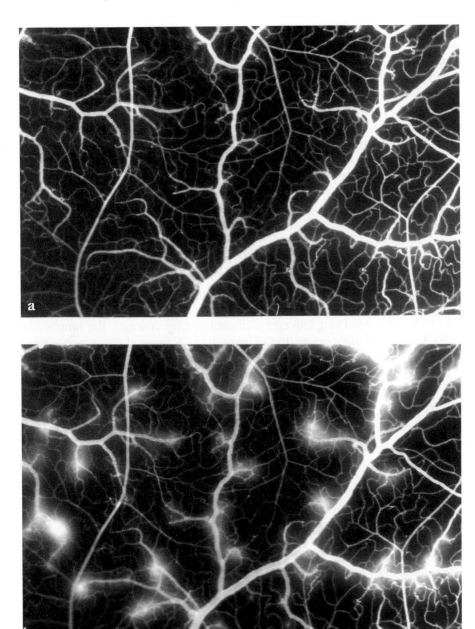

Figure 1. – Fluorescent micrograph of the hamster cheek pouch after i.v. injection of 150,000-dalton FITC-dextran. Same area before (a) and 5 min after (b) topical application of bradykinin 4 x 10^{-7} M for 5 min. Several leakage sites at postcapillary venules are shown by extravasation of FITC-dextran.

at a constant flow. The superfusion solution is fed into a cuvette of a fluorimeter for continuous measurements of FITC-dextran concentration. Properly dissected the hamster cheek pouch preparation gives excellent optical resolution and is an untraumatized preparation to judge from the presence of vascular tone (vasomotion) and the absence of FITC-dextran leakage sites or intravascular leukocyte accumulation for several hours.

Illumination of the preparation with a 100 W Hg lamp and filtering of the light for FITC-microscopy clearly reveal the intravascular FITC-dextran *(Figure 1 a)* and how FITC-dextran is leaking from postcapillary venules following topical application of bradykinin *(Figure 1 b)*.

In most preparations there is no visible extravasation of FITC-dextran (leakage sites) although the concentration of FITC-dextran in the superfusing buffer increases immediately (in less than 3 min) after its injection to reach a maximum around 30 minutes later. Preparations with no or fading leaks and no further increase in FITC-dextran concentration after 30 min are acceptable for experiments [18].

Autacoids and drugs that could affect macromolecular permeability can now be added to the superfusion buffer before it flows over the cheek pouch *(Table I)*. Microvascular leakage is quantitated by counting the number of leaks per cm^2 of the preparation *(Figure 1 b)*. A linear dose-response-rela-

Table I. – Mediators that increase FITC-dextran leakage in postcapillary venules (intravital microscopy)

Mediator	Effective conc., M
Histamine, serotonin	10^{-6}
Bradykinin, substance P	10^{-7}
ADP, adenosine, inosine	10^{-5}
Prostaglandins E_1, E_2, $F_{2\alpha}$	$>10^{-8}$
Leukotrienes C_4, D_4, E_4, B_4	$>10^{-9}$
Complement, C3a, C5a	$>10^{-9}$
Platelet activating factor (PAF)	$>10^{-9}$
Fibrin derived peptides	-
Free radicals, ischemia	-
Immune aggregates	-
Phorbol ester (PDBu)	10^{-6}
Oxidant injury (tertiar-butyl-hydroperoxid)	$4 \cdot 10^{-4}$
Endotoxin (E. coli 0111.B4)	(0.7 µg/ml)

tionship between the number of leaks and the logaritmic dose of bradykinin has been shown [7]. Several leukotrienes (LTC$_4$, LTD$_4$, LTA$_4$, LTB$_4$) and histamine also induce a linear dose-dependent increase in number of leaks [19]. The number of leaks per cm^2 correlated with the amount of FITC-dextran eliminated by the superfusing buffer during 30 min after stimulation with histamine [18] or LTB$_4$ [20]. All mediators or noxious agents tested so far *(Table I)* induced a reversible increase in the number of leaks and FITC-dextran concentration of the superfusate as exemplified for LTB$_4$ *(Figure 2)*.

Modulation of mediator-induced permeability increase

Pharmacological inhibition of mediator-induced leak formation was first shown with a β_2-receptor agonist, terbutaline (0.5mg/kg b.w.), which reduced the bradykinin response by 83 % (21). Since then the inhibitory effect of β_2-agonist has been further characterized by the use of several other mediators [12, 18, 22] listed in *Table II*. The selective β_2-receptor antagonist ICI 118 551 could effectively block the antipermeability effect of terbutaline [22]. The β_2-blocker potentiated the histamine response by 20 % suggesting that endothelial cells may be under some influence of endogenous catecholamines. The specificity of β_2-receptors in postcapillary venules was shown in experiments with the (-)- and (+)-forms of terbutaline given either locally or as i.v. injection. The (+)-form had no effect at concentrations or i.v. doses which were 100 times higher than the effective concentrations or i.v. doses of the (-)-form [22]. The selective inhibition of the mediator-induced permeability increase with the (-)-form has also been shown in the canine forelimb preparation [23].

Several clinically important glucocorticoids, e.g. budesonide, dexamethasone and methylprednisolone (MP), have been studied in the cheek pouch both on local administration and after i.v. injection. Local treatment with the glucocorticoids resulted in a 90 % reduction of the number of histamine-induced leaks, when the glucocorticoid treatment was given 60 min before the histamine challenge [24]. The effect had a slower onset compared with the effects seen with other anti-inflammatory drugs which suggests that glucocorticoids acted on endothelial hormonal receptor, nuclear uptake and release or synthesis of active proteins. Results on immunoaggregate-induced release of histamine also suggested that the anti-permeability effect of MP was induced through a direct action on the endothelium. This release was not affected by MP given 24 hours before ovalbumin challenge. However, MP-treated

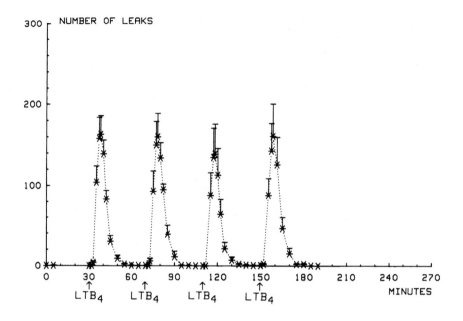

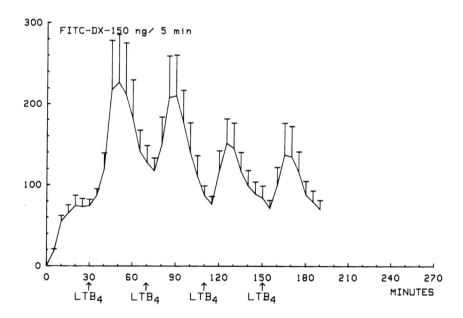

Figure 2. – The permeability increase in the number of leaks (top) and efflux of FITC-dextran (bottom) following four local applications of LTB_4 (10^{-8} M, 5 min) in 6 hamsters (mean ± SEM).

Table II. – Inhibitors of mediator-induced leakage of large molecules (FITC-dextran) in the hamster.

Inhibitor	Conc. M	Mediator
β_2-receptor agonist (terbutaline)	10^{-7}-10^{-6}	Histamine, bradykinin, ischemia, LTB_4 adenosine, phorbol ester, oxidant injury
Calcium antagonist (verapamil)	10^{-5}	Histamine, bradykinin
Glucocorticoids (budesonide, methyl-prednisolon, dexamethason)	10^{-7} (for 5 min) (10 mg/kg iv)	Histamine, bradykinin, LTB_4, LTC_4, PAF, immune agregate, ischemia, oxidant injury, phorbol ester, endotoxin
Theophylline	10^{-5}	Histamine
Vasopressin (and derivatives)	10^{-8}	Bradykinin, histamine
H_1-receptor antagonist (mepyramine)	10^{-5}	Histamine
$5HT_2$-receptor antagonist (ketanserin)	$5\cdot10^{-7}$	Serotonin, histamine
PKC-inhibitors H-7, staurosporin	10^{-5}-10^{-8}	Phorbol ester (Phorbol-12-13-dibutyrate, PDBu)
Superoxiddismutase (CuZn-SOD, EC-SOD)	(25 mg/kg iv)	Ischemia, oxidant injury

hamsters showed a reduced response to locally applied LTC_4, histamine and PAF-acether [25].

The fact that only 5 min of exposure was necessary for the glucocorticoids to exert a pronounced effect supports the hypothesis of a local effect on the endothelial cells in the postcapillary venules. As summarized in *Table II* such a short treatment effectively inhibits the action of several chemical mediators including endotoxin. However, the endotoxin-induced adhesion of leukocytes in the post-capillary venules was not reduced by budesonide, only the increase in vascular permeability was inhibited [26].

Phorbol ester (phorbol-12,13-dibutyrate = PDBu) is a potent stimulator of protein kinase C (PKC) and it induced leakage in postcapillary venules but unlike most other mediators *(Table I)* a marked tachyphylaxis was seen at a second PDBu-challenge several hours after the first [27]. Bradykinin stimulation after the two PDBu-applications gave a permeability increase within the normal range. Terbutaline and budesonide inhibited both PDBu and the bradykinin induced plasma leakage. Two putative PKC-inhibitors H-7 (an isoquinolinsulfonamid) and staurosporin inhibited the PDB_U but not the bradykinin induced response thus indicating a more selective inhibitory action than the β_2-receptor agonist and the glucocorticoid [27].

Conclusion

Some examples of pharmacological inhibition of mediator induced venular permeability (plasma leakage) have been presented. The mechanisms behind these antipermeability effects have to be different but at the present state of knowledge they might be explained as a result of direct actions on venular endothelial cells possibly involving relaxation of mediator-contracted endothelial cells.

References

1. Rotrosen D, Gallin JI. Histamine type I receptor occupancy increases endothelial cytosolic calcium, reduces F-actin, and promotes albumin diffusion across cultured endothelial monolayers. J Cell Biol 1986; 103 : 2379-2387.

2. Derian CK, Moskowitz MA. Polyphosphoinositide hydrolysis in endothelial cells and carotid artery segments. J Biol Chem 1986; 261 : 3831-3837.

3. Lambert TL, Kent RS, Whorton AR. Bradykinin stimulation of inositol polyphosphate production in porcine aortic endothelial cells. J Biol Chem 1986; 261 : 15288-15293.

4. Colden-Stanfield M, Schilling WP, Ritchie AK, *et al.* Bradykinin-induced increases in cytosolic calcium and ionic currents in cultured bovine aortic endothelial cells. Circ Rest 1987; 61 : 632-640.

5. Majno G, Palade GE. Studies on inflammation. I. The effect of histamine and serotonin on vascular permeability. An electron microscopic study. J Biophys Biochem Cytol 1961 ; 11 : 571.

6. Hultström D, Svensjö E. Intravital and electron microscopic study of bradykinin-induced vascular permeability changes using FITC-dextran as a tracer. J Pathol 1979, 129 : 125.

7. Svensjö E. Bradykinin and prostaglandin E_1, E_2 and $F_{2\alpha}$-induced macromolecular leakage in the hamster cheek pouch. Prostaglandines and Medicine 1978; 1 : 397-410.

8. Olesen S-P, Crone C. Substances that rapidly augment ionic conductance of endothelium in cerebral venules. Acta Physiol Scand 1986; 127 : 233-241.

9. Olesen S-P. Electrical resistance of arterioles and venules in the hamster cheek pouch. 1985; 123 : 121-126.

10. Simionescu N, Simionescu M, Palade GE. Open junctions in the endothelium of the postcapillary venules of the diaphragm. J Cell Biol 1978; 79 : 27.

11. Grega GJ, Svensjö E, Haddy FJ. Macromolecular permeability of the microvascular membrane : physiological and pharmacological regulation. Microcirculation 1981; 1 : 325-341.

12. Persson CGA, Svensjö E. Vascular responses and their suppression : drugs interfering with venular permeability. *In : Handbook of inflammation, Vol. 5, The pharmacology of inflammation.* Bonta IL, Bray MA, Parnham MJ, Eds, 1985, Amsterdam, Elsevier, pp 61-82.

13. Svensjö E, Grega GJ. Evidence for endothelial cell-mediated regulation of macromolecular permeability by postcapillary venules. Fed Proc 1986; 45 : 89-95.

14. Crone C. Modulation of solute permeability in microvascular endothelium. Federation Proc 1986; 45 : 77-83.

15. Svensjö E, Arfors K-E, Arturson G, *et al*. The hamster cheek pouch preparation as a model for studies of macromolecular permeability of the microvasculature. Uppsala J Med Sci 1978; 83 : 71-79.

16. Björk J, Smedegård G, Svensjö E, *et al*. The use of the hamster cheek pouch for intravital microscopy studies of microvascular events. Prog Appl Microcirc 1984; 6 : 41-53 (Karger, Basel).

17. Duling BR. The preparation and use of the hamster cheek pouch for studies of the microcirculation. Microvasc Res 1973; 5 : 423-429.

18. Svensjö E, Roempke K. Microvascular aspects on edema formation and its inhibition by β_2-receptor stimulants and some other antiinflammatory drugs. *In : Progress in Microcirculation research II* (CPME, Kensington, Australia), Garlick DG, Perry MA, Courtice FC, Eds, 1985.

19. Bjork J, Arfors KE, Dahlen SE, *et al*. Effects of leukotrienes on vascular permeability and leukocyte adhesion. 1981, *In : " The inflammatory process "*. P Venge and A Lindbom Eds, p. 103-112, Almqvist & Wiksell, Uppsala, Sweden.

20. Erlansson M, Svensjo E, Bergqvist D. Leukotriene B4-induced permeability increase in postcapillary venules and its inhibition by three different antiinflammatory drugs. Inflammation 1989; 13 : 693-705.

21. Svensjö E, Persson CGA, Rutili G. Inhibition of bradykinin induced macromolecular leakage from postcapillary venules by a β2-adrenoceptor stimulant, terbutaline. Acta Physiol Scandl 1977; 101 : 504-506.

22. Svensjö E, Roempke K. Dose-related antipermeability effect of terbutaline and its inhibition by a selective β_2-receptor blocking agent. Agents and Actions 1985; 16 : (1/2), 19-20.

23. Dobbins DE, Buehn MJ, Dabney JM. Bradykinin-mediated edema formation is blocked by levorotatory but not dextrorotatory terbutaline. Microcirc Endoth Lymphatics 1988; 5 : 377-397.

24. Svensjö E, Roempke K. Time-dependent inhibition of bradykinin-induced microvascular permeability increase by local glucocorticoid treatment. Respiration 1984; 46 : (Suppl. 1), 60.

25. Bjork J, Goldschmidt T, Smedegard G, *et al*. Methylprednisolone acts at the endothelial cell level reducing inflammatory responses. Acta Physiol Scand 1985, 123 : 221-224.

26. Svensjö E, Erlansson M, Van den Bos GC. Endotoxininduced increase in leukocyte adherence and macromolecular permeability of postcapillary venules. Agents and Actions 1990; 29 : 21-23.

27. Svensjö E, Roempke K. Inhibition of phorbol ester induced microvascular leakage by a putative protein kinase C inhibitor, terbutaline and budesonide. Int J Microcirc 1988; 7 : p. 85 (abstract).

Return circulation and Norepinephrine : an update. Ed. P.M. Vanhoutte. John Libbey Eurotext, Paris © 1991, pp. 207-218.

21

Microcirculatory responses to *Ruscus* extract in the hamster cheek pouch

E. Bouskela

Department of Physiology and Biophysics, University of Lund, Sölvegatan 19, S-223 62, Lund, Sweden

Introduction

Ruscus aculeatus is a very common plant, growing in all temperate regions of the world. The hydroalcoholic extract of its roots is used for the treatment of venous insufficiency, alone or in combination with other compounds [2, 3, 12]. The mechanisms of action proposed for *Ruscus* extract are (a) direct activation of postjunctional α1 and α2 adrenergic receptors and (b) displacement of stored norepinephrine from adrenergic nerve endings [8]. These activities have been demonstrated on veins and lymph vessels [7, 9, 10]. The present study was undertaken to determine the effects of *Ruscus* extract upon the microcirculation of the hamster cheek pouch (*in vivo* preparation). To our knowledge, there are no data available in the literature on the effects of this extract upon arterioles and venules, at the microcirculatory level. The routes used for administration of *Ruscus* extract, in this study, were oral, intravenous and topical. When topical application was studied, experiments were performed at different temperatures : 25 °C, 36.5°C and 40 °C.

Materials and Methods

For oral administration of *Ruscus* extract, twelve male hamsters, 7 to 10 weeks old, weight range from 75 to 120 g, were housed in individual cages and divided in two groups, R and W, 6 animals in each group. The animals received either 0.2 ml of *Ruscus* extract solution [(150 mg/kg), group R] or 0.2 ml of water (group W) daily, always in the morning, for 28 days. Every animal was observed at the microscope on the 29th day after the onset of the oral administration.

For intravenous and topical administration of *Ruscus* extract, experiments were also performed on male hamsters, 7 to 10 weeks old, weight range from 75 to 120 g.

Anesthesia was induced by an intraperitoneal injection of 0.1-0.2 ml of sodium pentobarbital (Mebumal vet., 60 mg/ml) and maintained with α-chloralose (100 mg/kg) administered intravenously. The femoral artery and vein were cannulated for pressure measurements, anesthetic and *Ruscus* extract injections. Throughout the surgery and subsequent experiment, the animal rested on a heating pad controlled by a rectal thermistor and body temperature was maintained at 36.5°C. A tracheal tube was inserted to facilitate spontaneous breathing. The hamster was placed on a stage containing a chamber with a silicon rubber ring surrounding a transillumination window. This chamber was preceded by another one which pre-heated the superfusion solution. Both chambers were mounted with Peltier elements for temperature control, allowing easy change and regulation of the superfusate's temperature. The cheek pouch was carefully everted with the aid of a moist cotton stick and the distal, non-muscular, part of it identified and pinned to a silicon ring [1, 13]. Dissection was performed under a stereomicroscope : a crescent-shaped incision was made in the top layer, the flap was pinned to the side and the areolar connective tissue removed to expose the bottom layer vasculature for microscopic observations. During the preparation and throughout the experiment, the cheek pouch was constantly superfused with a bicarbonate buffered saline solution (NaCl 131.9 mM ; KCl 4.7 mM ; $CaCl_2.2H_2O$ 2.0 mM ; $MgSO_4.7H_2O$ 1.2 mM and $NaHCO_3$ 20.0 mM) at a rate of 4.6 ml/ min. This solution was continuously bubbled with 5 % CO_2 in N_2. This gas mixture was also continuously blowed through a perforated ring located on top of the transillumination window to assure that PO_2 in the superfusion solution bathing the pouch was maintained lower than 15 mmHg.

An intravital videomicroscope was used to observe the microcirculation and make microcirculatory measurement. The total magnification of the video image was 1000X. The TV monitor display was used to obtain arteriolar and venular diameter measurements by an image shearing monitor, IPM, model

907. During the whole experimental period, the diameter of arterioles and venules were recorded on videotape. In practice, we used videotape replay for final determination of vessel diameters, since greater attention could be given to this measurement than was possible during the conduct of the experiment. These measurements were recorded in a 6-channel stripchart record (Grass polygraph model RCS7C8).

For the oral administration part of the study, the experimental protocol consisted of sets of measurements performed on the same region in every animal. A venule with two side branches (collecting venules) and an arteriole with two side branches were measured in each preparation.

For the systemic IV administration part of the study, the experimental protocol consisted of sets of measurements performed every 10 min, exactly on the same site. During each set, data on vessel internal diameter as well as on arterial pressure were collected. The first 3 sets constituted the control period. After it, *Ruscus* extract, 5 mg/kg, was injected intravenously. The measurements started immediately after the injection and were performed every 10 min for 60 min.

For the topical administration part of the study, the experimental protocol consisted of sets of measurements performed exactly at the same site before and after different concentrations of *Ruscus* extract had been added to the superfusate. One to four arterioles and venules were studied in each animal. Six different concentrations of *Ruscus* extract were tested in every preparation : 5.10^{-3}, 10.10^{-3}, 50.10^{-3}, 100.10^{-3}, 500.10^{-3} and 1000.10^{-3} mg/ml. The animals were divided in three groups, depending on the temperature the cheek pouch was maintained during the experiment : Group I, 36.5°C ; Group II, 25.0°C and Group III, 40.0°C.

The results are expressed as either mean ± S.D., mean ± S.E.M. or ranges. Statistical significances were determined by the use of Student's t test and probabilities of less than 5 % (P<0.05) were considered significant.

Results

Oral administration

The animals were weighed once a week and there was no significant difference between the two groups *(Table I and Figure 1)*.

One animal of each group had problems during the surgical procedure and died.

Table I. – Body weight (g) of male hamsters receiving either *Ruscus* extract (group R) or water (group W)

Group	Day 0	Day 7	Day 14	Day 21	Day 28
R	90.0	90.0	95.5	93.4	95.9
R	100.0	100.0	115.3	113.5	114.5
R	95.0	100.0	108.1	110.0	112.6
R	100.0	100.0	113.2	114.0	113.7
R	85.0	85.0	87.1	85.2	88.5
R	85.0	90.0	94.1	97.4	93.7
W	90.0	95.0	106.8	107.2	107.4
W	95.0	95.0	103.6	106.2	108.7
W	100.0	100.0	105.7	107.0	108.2
W	80.0	80.0	82.8	84.7	87.0
W	90.0	90.0	97.1	100.2	102.5
W	80.0	85.0	94.1	94.7	92.9

Day 0 = onset of the oral administration

Table II. – Oral administration of *Ruscus* extract. Internal diameter (μm) of venules (V), venular side branches (SV), arterioles (A) and arteriolar side branches (SA).

Vessel type	Group R	Group W
V	42.82±3.28* (5)	60.76±6.80 (5)
SV	23.45±2.77 (10)	29.28±2.48 (10)
A	30.58±3.43* (5)	22.22±4.80 (5)
SA	14.77±0.86 (10)	13.78±1.25 (10)

Mean ± S.E.M.

(n)

* Significantly different from control (group W)

210

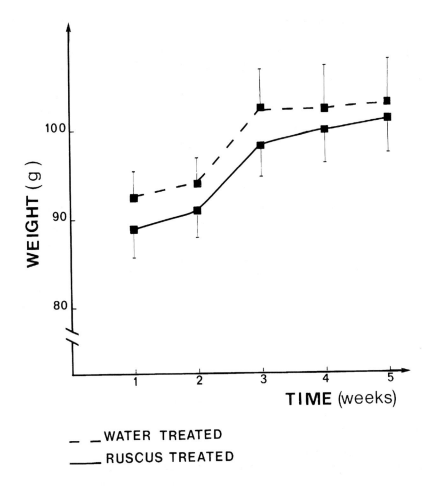

Figure 1. – Body weight of hamsters receiving either *Ruscus* extract or water (oral administration). Each point indicates mean ± S.E.M.

Mean arterial pressure was 95 ± 4 mmHg (mean ± S.E.M.) for the R group and 93 ± 7 mmHg for the W group.

The diameter of the studied vessels ranged from a) 35.0 to 85.4 µm for the venules; b) 10.9 to 42.8 µm for the venular side branches; c) 14.8 to 38.6 µm for the arterioles and d) 9.6 to 20.5 µm for the arteriolar side branches.

Oral administration of *Ruscus* extract (150 mg/kg during 28 days) elicited a 30 % constriction of the studied venules and a 37 % dilatation of the arterioles. The arteriolar and venular side branches were not affected *(Table II)*.

211

Systemic IV administration

Studies were performed on 7 male hamsters, weighing 97.6±6.1 g (mean ± S.E.M.). Arterioles, diameter range 10.0 to 35.0 μm and venules, diameter range 15.0 to 63.0 μm, were observed. *Table III* summarizes the results obtained.

Systemic intravenous administration of *Ruscus* extract, 5 mg/kg, provoked venular constriction and did not affect the arteriolar diameter in any considerable degree *(Table III and Figure 2)*. Mean arterial pressure was not affected by the intravenous injection of *Ruscus* extract in the dose used.

Topical administration

Studies were performed on 18 male hamsters, weighing 95.0±9.1 g (mean ± S.D.).

Arterioles, diameter range 11.7 to 74.9 μm and venules, diameter range 23.3 to 134.5 μm, were observed. *Tables IV, V* and *VI* show the results obtained at 36.5°C, 25.0°C and 40.0°C, respectively. The effects of topical application of different concentrations of *Ruscus* extract on arterioles and venules depended upon the temperature in which the hamster cheek pouch preparation was observed *(Figures 3 and 4)*. At 25.0°C, arterioles and venules dilated. At 36.5°C, arterioles either dilated for topical concentrations up to 50.10^{-3} mg/ml of *Ruscus* extract or remained unchanged when higher concentrations were applied, while the venules constricted. At 40.0°C, arterioles either did not change diameter for topical concentrations up to 10.10^{-3} mg/ml of the

Table III. – Intravenous administration (5 mg/kg) of *Ruscus* extract. Internal diameter of arterioles (A) and venules (V).

After	10 min	20 min	30 min	40 min	50 min	60 min
V 89.82±2.92*	92.99±1.61*	92.27±1.57	93.93±2.41*	90.66±5.05	90.16±3.13*	94.34±2.66*
(24)	(16)	(15)	(18)	(10)	(15)	(16)
A 100.30±2.14	96.42±1.81	98.94±3.03	100.52±3.64	102.13±3.05	98.74±3.79	95.30±3.35
(17)	(10)	(13)	(10)	(11)	(10)	(10)

To facilitate the comparison, the values are expressed as percentage of control dimensions. Mean ± S.E.M.
(n)
* Significantly different from control ($P<0.05$).

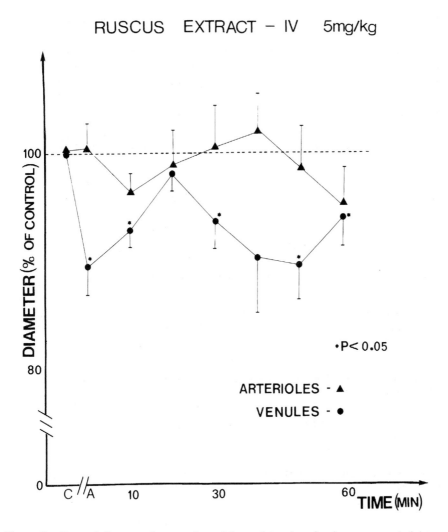

Figure 2. – Internal diameter changes of arterioles and venules after intravenous administration of *Ruscus* extract (5 mg/kg). To facilitate the comparison, the values are expressed as percentage of control dimensions. Each point indicates mean ± S.E.M.

extract or constricted when higher concentrations were applied, while the venules constricted.

Mean arterial pressure and the temperature of the animal were not affected by the experimental procedures.

Table IV. – Topical administration of *Ruscus* extract. Hamster cheek pouch microcirculation at 36.5°C

	Concentration of *Ruscus extract (mg/ml)*		
	5.10^{-3}	10.10^{-3}	50.10^{-3}
Arterioles	113.54±5.98	113.60±6.23	103.98±2.68
	(8)	(8)	(8)
Venules	95.94±2.40	95.46±2.18	92.30±2.23*
	(13)	(13)	(19)
	100.10^{-3}	500.10^{-3}	1000.10^{-3}
Arterioles	100.32±3.36	102.77±3.87	102.66±4.96
	(11)	(11)	(11)
Venules	92.28±2.01*	88.85±1.31*	88.64±2.48*
	(19)	(19)	(19)

To facilitate the comparison, the values are expressed as percentage of control dimensions.
Mean ± S.E.
(n)
* Significantly different from control

Table V. – Topical administration of *Ruscus* extract. Hamster cheek pouch microcirculation at 25.0°C

	Concentration of *Ruscus* extract (mg/ml)		
	5.10^{-3}	10.10^{-3}	50.10^{-3}
Arterioles	108.08±2.54*	111.65±3.37*	113.10±3.72*
	(11)	(11)	(11)
Venules	104.35±3.66	106.94±2.76*†	105.47±3.42†
	(22)	(22)	(22)
	100.10^{-3}	500.10^{-3}	1000.10^{-3}
Arterioles	118.58±2.75*†	118.03±2.94*†	111.03±4.92*
	(11)	(11)	(11)
Venules	108.07±2.87*†	106.73±2.82*†	111.67±2.65*†
	(22)	(22)	(22)

To facilitate the comparison, the values are expressed as percentage of control dimensions.
Mean ± S.E.
(n)
* Significantly different from control (P<0.05)
† Significantly different from the 36.5°C value

Table VI. – Topical administration of *Ruscus* extract. Hamster cheek pouch microcirculation at 40.0°C.

	Concentration of *Ruscus* extract (mg/ml)		
	5.10^{-3}	10.10^{-3}	50.10^{-3}
Arterioles	103.64±1.53	102.93±2.19	97.00±1.68†
	(12)	(12)	(12)
Venules	93.32±0.71*	90.24±0.72*†	85.50±1.28*†
	(20)	(20)	(20)
	100.10^{-3}	500.10^{-3}	1000.10^{-3}
Arterioles	94.00±2.02*	87.97±1.23*†	84.32±0.97*†
	(12)	(12)	(12)
Venules	82.39±1.57*†	77.73±1.86*†	75.70±1.86*†
	(20)	(20)	(20)

To facilitate the comparison, the values are expressed as percentage of control dimension

Mean S.E.

(n)

* = significantly different from control (P<0.05)

† = significantly different from the 36.5°C value

Discussion

Several studies have demonstrated that *Ruscus* extract improves venous insufficiency. Rudofsky [11] reported a decrease of approximately 10 % in venous capacity 2h after oral administration of *Ruscus* extract in healthy volunteers.

Patients suffering from chronic venous insufficiency, treated with *Ruscus* extract, maintained a constant venous tone and improved venous emptying, unlike placebo patients [6]. In isolated canine saphenous veins, the extract of the roots of *Ruscus aculeatus* caused contractions [9]. Rubanyi *et al.* [10] showed that local warming augmented the venoconstriction evoked by *Ruscus* extract possibly because it facilitated the α1 adrenergic component of the venous smooth muscle response to the extract. Moderate cooling (from 37°C to 24°C) affects α-adrenergic contractile responses in canine cutaneous and deep veins differently [4]. By cooling, contractile responses to norepinephrine or sympathetic nerve stimulation are augmented in cutaneous veins

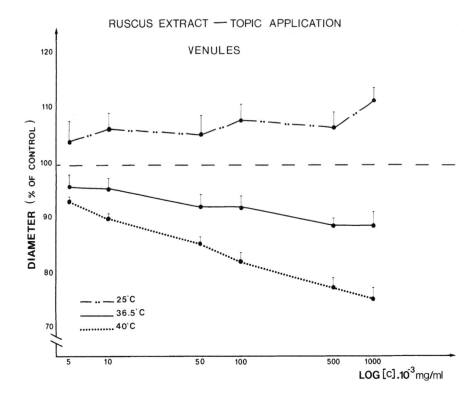

Figure 3. – Internal diameter changes of venules after topical application of different concentrations of *Ruscus* extract. Experiments were performed at 25.0°C, 36.5°C and 40.0°C. To facilitate the comparison, the values are expressed as percentage of control dimensions. Each point indicates mean ± S.E.M.

and depressed in the deep ones. In rings of saphenous veins, from control rabbits, *Ruscus* extract evoked concentration dependent contractions which were insensitive to prazosin and rauwolscine [5]. Cooling augmented these contractions and warming caused an increase in tone.

In our study, oral administration of *Ruscus* extract elicited a 30 % constriction of venules with internal diameter larger than 35 µm. The smaller venules were not affected. These findings could be explained by (a) lack of well defined smooth muscle layer and/or (b) lack of nerve endings in the smaller venules.

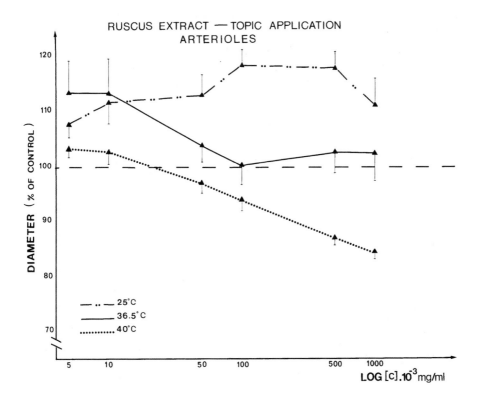

Figure 4. – Internal diameter changes of arterioles after topical application of different concentrations of *Ruscus* extract. Experiments were performed at 25.0°C, 36.5°C and 40.0°C. To facilitate the comparison, the values are expressed as percentage of control dimensions. Each point indicates mean ± S.E.M.

Systemic intravenous administration of *Ruscus* extract evoked venular constriction and did not affect the arteriolar diameter.

Topical application of *Ruscus* extract elicited concentration and temperature dependent responses in the studied vessels. At 25.0°C, arterioles and venules dilated ; at 36.5°C, arterioles dilated or remained unchanged depending on the concentration used, while the venules constricted and at 40.0°C, arterioles remained unchanged or constricted depending on the concentration used while the venules constricted.

The observed differences between the responses of arterioles and venules after *Ruscus* extract administration could be explained by an augmented liberation of endothelium-derived relaxing factor on the arteriolar side (Miller *et al.*, this volume).

In conclusion, the effects of *Ruscus* extract observed *in vivo,* at microcirculatory level, are in agreement with the data previously reported in the literature on larger blood vessels and in patients with venous insufficiency.

Acknowledgements

The author wishes to thank Pierre Fabre Medicament for the generous supply of *Ruscus* extract. The skillful assistance of Ms. Fatima Z.G.A. Cyrino is also gratefully acknowledged.

References

1. Duling BR. The preparation and use of the hamster cheek pouch for studies of the microcirculation. Microvasc Res 1973; 5:423-429.
2. Elbaz C, Nebot F, Reinharez D. Insuffisance veineuse des membres inférieurs. Etude contrôlée de l'action du Cyclo 3. Phlébologie 1976; 29 (1):77-84.
3. Fayolle J. Cyclo 3: Indications thérapeutiques actuelles en phlébologie médicale. Cah Méd Lyonnais 1970; 46:1497-1498.
4. Flavahan NA, Vanhoutte PM Thermosensitivity of cutaneous and deep veins. Phlebology 1988; 3 (suppl. 1): 41-45.
5. Harker CT, Marcelon G, Vanhoutte PM. Temperature, oestrogens and contractions of venous smooth muscle of the rabbit. Phlebology 1988; 3 (suppl. 1):77-82.
6. Lozes A, Boccalon H. Double blind study of *Ruscus* extract: venous plethysmographic results in man. Inter Angio 1984; 3:99-102.
7. Marcelon G, Pouget G, Tisne-Versailles J. Effect of *Ruscus* on the adrenoceptors of the canine lymphatic thoracic duct. Phlebology 1988; 3 (suppl. 1):109-112.
8. Marcelon G, Vanhoutte PM. Mechanisms of action of *Ruscus* extract. Inter Angio 1984; 3:74-76.
9. Marcelon G, Verbeuren TJ, Lauressergues H, *et al.* Effect of *Ruscus aculeatus* on isolated canine cutaneous veins. Gen Pharmac 1983; 14:103-106.
10. Rubanyi G, Marcelon G, Vanhoutte PM. Effect of temperature on the responsiveness of cutaneous veins to the extract of *Ruscus aculeatus.* Gen Pharmac 1984; 15:431-434.
11. Rudofsky G. Plethysmographic studies of venous capacity and venous outflow and venotropic therapy. Inter Angio 1984; 3:95-98.
12. Sicard P. Resultats avec Cyclo 3 dans le traitement des ulcères variqueux. Phlébologie 1971; 1:117-121.
13. Svensjö E, Arfors KE, Arturson G. *et al.* The hamster cheek pouch preparation as a model for studies of macromolecular permeability of the microvasculaire. Uppsala J Med Sci 1978; 83:71-79.

Return circulation and Norepinephrine : an update. Ed. P.M. Vanhoutte. John Libbey Eurotext, Paris © 1991, pp. 219-224.

22

Effect of *Ruscus* extract*
on the capillary filtration rate

G. Rudofsky

*Angiology Clinic and Polyclinic, Essen University Hospital,
Hufelandstraße 55, 4300 Essen 1, Germany*

The causal chain consisting of insufficient venous valves, inadequate venous blood removal with venous hypervolaemia, a resultant insufficient drop in pressure, and a rise in pressure in the capillaries producing dilation of the capillaries ultimately leads to microcirculation disturbances due to the retardation of perfusion, increased filtration of liquid, and exsudation of protein into tissue, and thus to the formation of edemas [4].

As damaged venous valves cannot be restored and intact valves in dilated varicose veins are no longer capable of closing, attempts are made to compensate for the increased venous pressure by applying external pressure with dressings or compression stockings, to increase the tissue pressure and at the same time to reduce the elevated filtration rate using capillary-sealing drugs.

Ruscus extract and trimethylhesperidin chalcone [3] have been shown to act on the filtration rate in various animal experiments and clinical studies [1-5]. However, it has been demonstrated in experimental clinical studies that different filtration rates were measured, depending on the group concerned. Thus, the change in capillary permeability produced by *Ruscus* extract in

---

* Phlebodril®

healthy volunteers with a venous capacity of 4.8 ml/100ml tissue was about 0.3 ml/min, whereas in volunteers with a venous capacity of 3.5 ml/100 ml tissue a change of only 0.1 ml/min was found. It therefore seemed reasonable to assume that the filtration rate measurable by plethysmography may be influenced by various physical characteristics.

To check this hypothesis a meta-analysis was therefore made of three studies with similar designs, to investigate the effect of various factors such as age, sex, weight and height, and venous capacity on the filtration rate.

Material and methods

Baseline data

Each of the three studies was performed as a randomized double-blind cross-over. In the first two studies healthy volunteers were investigated, receiving 450 mg *Ruscus* extract and 450 mg trimethylhesperidin chalcone (TMHC) as a single dose or 184 mg *Ruscus* extract together with 184 mg melilot extract applied topically. In the third study female patients with CVI stage I received 6g cream (96 mg *Ruscus* extract and 96 mg melilot extract) as a single dose.

Method

The action of the test substances on capillary permeability was determined in the three studies with the same apparatus (Gutmann Periquant), using the increase or decrease in tissue volume and venous occlusion plethysmography in a standard procedure [7]. The occlusion time was 10 min, with a occlusion pressure of 80 mm Hg. The rise in volume between the 5th and 10th minutes of congestion was taken to be the filtration rate.

Evaluation

The effect of the various physical characteristics, venous capacity, dosage form, and diagnosis (healthy - CVI) on the filtration rate was at first examined in a stepwise, multiple linear regression. In each case the values measured before administration of the drugs in the three studies were used as the reference level.

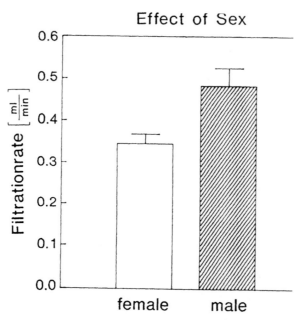

Figure 1. – Filtration rate of healthy volunteers; mean (x) and standard error (SE).

To demonstrate the action of the drugs, the factors identified as significant were then used as covariates in an analysis of variance (repeated measure design).

Results

The following correlations were identified in the regression calculation :
The filtration rate was not affected by age (p>0.10). Men have a filtration rate distinctly higher than women (p = 0.07) *(Figure 1)*. The filtration rate shows a significant drop with increasing Broca index (p = 0.005) *(Figure 2)*. As expected, in patients with CVI the filtration rate was clearly higher than in healthy volunteers (p = 0.033). The greatest correlation was found between the venous capacity and filtration rate (p < 0.001) *(Figure 3)*.

After adjusting the filtration rate for these factors, a highly significant treatment effect was found (p < 0.001). Within 2 h of the administration of *Ruscus* extract the filtration rate dropped by 0.17 ml/min *(Figure 4)*. This means

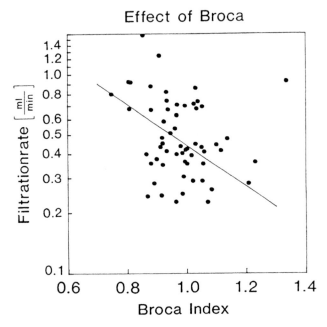

Figure 2. – Effect of Broca Index on filtration rate; n = 60.

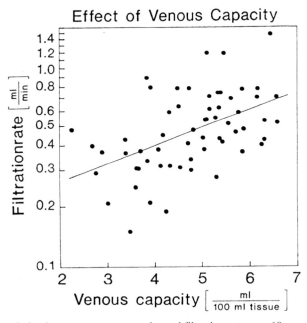

Figure 3. – Correlation between venous capacity and filtration rate; n = 60.

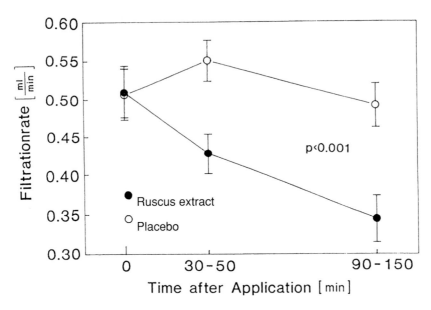

Figure 4. – Effect of treatment with *Ruscus* extract on filtration rate mean (x) and standard error (SE). The slopes of the curves differ significantly.

a decrease of 33 % referred to the baseline value of 0.51 ml/min. The duration of action was clearly longer than 2 h.

Discussion

The results show that *Ruscus* extract can exert a lasting effect on increased capillary permeability, one of the principal causes of microcirculation disturbance. The second characteristic of *Ruscus* extract, the tonic effect, has been demonstrated in animal experiments [12] and in clinical studies in healthy volunteers [3-5] and in patients [11]. Given the close connection between filtration rate and venous capacity, it could be assumed that a reduction in capillary filtration is achieved merely by increasing venous tone. This would mean that the same drug effect, i.e. the increase in venous tone, was measured by two different methods. However the highly significant effect of treatment on the capillary filtration rate after adjustment for the effect of venous capacity shows that the increase in venous tone and the reduction in capillary filtration are separate effects, but that both are produced by *Ruscus* extract in combination with TMHC or melilot extract.

This edema-protective effect is also supported by an improvement in lymph drainage. Thus, the lymphokinetic action of flavonoids and coumarin has been known for a long time [8, 9]. Animal studies demonstrate that the α-adrenergic action of *Ruscus* extract increased the motricity of the lymph vessels [10].

The interaction between capillary sealing and the increase in lymph flow should therefore produce a clear reduction in patients with venous edema congestion caused by chronic venous insufficiency, irrespective of its etiology. This has been demonstrated in a multicentre study with 141 patients [11].

References

1. Felix W, Nieberle J, Schmidt G. Protektive Wirkung von Trimethylhesperidinchalkon und *Ruscus aculeatus* genenüber Etacrynsäureödem am Hinterlauf der narkotisierten Katze. Phlebol Proktol 1983; 12 : 209-218.

2. Hönig I, Felix W. Effect on the permeability of isolated ear vein of the pig; a comparison between flavonoids and saponins. *In : Phlebologie' 89*. Davy A., Stemmer R. (eds), John Libbey Eurotext 680-682, London 1989.

3. Rudofsky G, Hirche H. Plethysmographische Untersuchungen eines Venentherapeutikums bei wärmebedingten hämodynamischen Veränderungen. Med Welt 1985; 36 : 145-149.

4. Rudofsky G. Venentonisierung und Kapillarabdichtung. Fort Med 107; (19) 430-434.

5. Rudofsky G. Transkutane Venentonisierung und Kapillarabdichtung bei gesunden Probanden. MMW 1989; 131 : (18) 362-365.

6. Schnitzer W, Klatt J, Baeker H, *et al.* Vergleich von szintigraphischen und plethysmographischen Messungen zur Bestimmung des kapillaren Filtrationskoeffizienten in der menschlichen Extremität. Basic Res Cardiol 1978; 73 : 77-84.

7. Rudofsky G, Esch P, Moser S, Ein Beitrag zur Standardisierung der Venenkapazitätsmessung. Act Chir 1984; 19 : 86-88.

8. Estler CJ. Zur Pharmakologie der Bioflavonoide. Fortschr Med 1971; 89 : 669-617.

9. Casley-Smith JR, Casley Smith Judith R. High protein œdemas and the benzopyrones. Lippincott Sydney, 1986.

10. Marcelon G, Pouget G, Tisné-Versailles J. Effect of *Ruscus* on the adrenoceptors of canine lymphatic thoracic duct. Phlebology 1988; 3 : (Suppl. 1) 109-112.

11. Rudofsky G, Diehm C, Gruß J, *et al.* Wirksamkeit einer Kombination venoaktiver Substanzen bei Patienten mit chronisch venöser Insuffizienz im Stadium I. *In : Therapie der Venener-krankungen*, Denck H., van Dongen R.J.A.M. (eds) 73-92, TM-Verlag, Hameln 1989.

12. Marcelon G, Vanhoutte PM. Venotonic effect of *Ruscus* under variable temperature conditions *in vitro*. Phlebology 1988; 3 : Suppl. 1, 51-54.

Return circulation and Norepinephrine : an update. Ed. P.M. Vanhoutte. John Libbey Eurotext, Paris © 1991, pp. 225-236.

23

Hemorheological concepts in venous insufficiency and implications for treatment with *Ruscus* extract*

C. Le Devehat, T. Khodabandehlou, M. Vimeux, G. Bondoux

Unité de Recherches d'Hémorhéologie clinique, Centre Hospitalier de Nevers, Centre de Diabétologie, 58320 Pougues-les-Eaux, France

Introduction

The disturbances in rheological properties of the blood are of interest as a possible pathological mechanism of venous stasis and thrombosis. Also of clinical importance is the possibility of hemorheologically oriented treatment of venous insufficiency. The albumin/fibrinogen ratio not only largely determines the viscosity of the plasma, but also affects the whole blood viscosity at low shear rates as the principal factor causing red cell aggregation. In contrast, red cell aggregability is thought to be the principal reason for the increased viscosity of the whole blood at low flow rates. The microrheological changes would thus be both a consequence and a cause of the venous stasis on the post capillary venular compartment. When there is a venous stasis, the red cell aggregates persist because the prevailing local flow forces are

---

*Cyclo-3 Fort

not adequate for their fluid dynamic dispersal. In venous stasis, blood is characterized by disturbances of thixotropy or structural viscosity, that is the increase in viscosity due to retarded flow. Drugs' action upon the red cell aggregation are to be considered as additional useful treatment in patients with venous insufficiency. Thus, in order to explain and confirm the clinical interest of *Ruscus* extract as a treatment for venous insufficiency, a preliminary study in a double blind test with placebo was carried out on 25 patients with venous insufficiency of the lower limbs with varicose.

State of art in microcirculation

The microrheological parameters that determine blood viscosity have an important physiological and physiopathological contribution to the understanding and the treatment of vascular pathologies. Venous pathology is characterized by a relative incapacity of the venous system to return back to the heart. Even if valvular incompetence is its basic etiology, numerous studies have shown that the phenomenon of venous insufficiency also is the result of modifications to the vascular wall and especially of important disturbances in the rheological properties of the blood [1]. The essential characteristic of blood viscosity is its increase in vascular sites where the flow is slowed down. In the veins, in the physiological state, the shear rates are the lowest and stasis phenomena can carry very important hyperpressures. Equally, with veins, the shear stress threshold is more elevated, all the more that the blood circulation is stationary. The microrheological parameters play a determining role in the phenomena of cellular activation and aggregation and also in the appearance of a local ischemia or thrombosis. In venous stasis, the venous blood flow is characterized by an increase in viscosity [2]. If, in vascular sites with high blood flow or high shear rates, the deformability of red cells is the determinant of blood viscosity, in contrast, in vascular sites with low flow or low shear rates, blood viscosity is primarily dependent on the aggregation-disaggregation phenomenon of red cells. These two phenomena of aggregation-disaggregation and of deformability of red cells are the microrheological factors controlling the fundamental processes in hemorheology [3, 4]. The degree of deformation of the red cell depends on exterior forces that act on this red cell and on its intrinsic rheological properties. Since the studies of Fahreus in 1921 on erythrocyte aggregates known as "rouleaux", we know that the formation of cellular structures depends, at the same time, on the plasma proteins (eg. fibrinogen [5, 6]), on the local hematocrit, on the erythrocyte deformability, on the aggregation tendency and on the conditions of blood flow [7]. Erythrocyte aggregation results, from the interactions between deformable particles, red cells and from the center of a fluid carrier, the plasma. Every outside or inside cause susceptible of modifying these interactions will have an influence on aggregation and will govern the viscoelastic behavior or different *thixotropics* [3, 8]. In venous insufficiency, where the blood flow is low, when the shear rate and the shear stress are insufficient, the blood viscosity increases primarily because of the aggregation of red cells which, by an intercellular link of fibrinogen and of plasma globulins, arrange themselves in a network of aggregates which are more or less dissociable [2, 3, 5-7]. The measurement of microrheological parameters is essential for studies concerning pathological circumstances characterized by a hyperviscosity syndrome.

The increase of blood viscosity associated with an elevated incidence of venous thrombosis in vascular varicose vein patients tends to confirm for the clinician that hemorheological disturbances participate largely in the genesis of venous thrombosis [9, 10]. Thus, in these areas of stasis where blood flow is very low and where rheological abnormalities are major, the consequence can result in a decrease of oxygen pressure and in the accumulation of toxic cellular metabolites (ADP, free radicals). From a physiopathological point of view, the appearance and prolongation in time and space of an hyperviscosity syndrome, even local, entails rheological modifications : the capacity of the red blood cells to the carried by the axial current disappears, the aggregates are formed, these disturb the conditions of blood flow which may result in the cessation of flow, of lesions on the tissue by anoxia and finally in thrombosis [11, 12]. In veins, where the rate of blood flow is the lowest and where a stasis is frequent at the time of varicose veins, erythrocyte aggregation appears as the fundamental parameter in the comprehension of rheological abnormalities of blood. All the more, the aggregation is controlled by numerous factors such as shear rate, hematocrit, intrinsic properties of erythrocytes, fibrinogen and the chemical or physical properties of the environment. An excess of local aggregation or an increase of the threshold of disaggregation leads the appearance of pathological aggregates [13, 14], by the formation of inter-erythrocytary links of fibrinogen [7, 15, 16]. Hematocrit, fibrinogen level, plasma viscosity and increased aggregation index of red cells, in situations of circulation at low shear rate, diminish the transport of oxygen leading to a relative hypoxia. This, aggravated by a decrease in erythrocyte deformability, influences equally the exchange of transcapillary liquids. In fact, the preferential increase of post-capillary resistance which results in these disturbances, in relation to precapillary resistance, elevates capillary pressure to a transcapillary passage of liquid provoking hemoconcentration, tissular œdema, an acidosis and a liberation and accumulation of aggregates and toxic substances.

Material and methods

A double blind test against placebo, was carried out on 45 subjects : 20 control subjects, 25 patients – 13 receiving the *Ruscus* extract in doses of 2 pills per day, in 2 doses, and 12 receiving a placebo.

Population

The 20 control subjects had no venous insufficiency, and were without medical treatment, without oral contraceptives and within the 95 % range of the ideal weight, according to the International Committee for Standardization in Haematology [17]. All had a packed cell volume (PCV) and erythrocyte indices, mean cell volume (MCV) and mean cell hemoglobin concentration (Mc Hc) within the normal range.

The 25 subjects suffering from venous insufficiency were characterized by varicose vein of the lower limbs, non smokers, without metabolic disease, with no history of previous thrombosis disease, without medical treatment or oral contraception.

Microrheological parameters

The hematocrit was measured by microcentrifugation at 12 500 g for 5 minutes (1/1) ; plasma fibrinogen (g/l) was determined by using a thrombin clotting time technique [18]; plasma viscosity (mPa.s) was measured at 37°C by a KSPV4 capillary viscometer [19]; red cell deformability was evaluated by filtration measurements using an initial flow rate method as described by Hanss [20]. This method consists of the filtration of a diluted red cell suspension in buffer medium through nucleopore polycarbonate sieves with 5 µ diameter pores. The red cell aggregation phenomenon was quantified by the Sefam erythroaggregameter [21]. This device consists of an automatic Couette viscometer. The blood suspensions, placed in a narrow gap between two co-axial cylinders and lightened by a laser beam, are subjected to a high shear rate (600 s-1) leading to a complete disaggregation of red cells. The shear rate, which is suddenly stopped, allows the "rouleaux" formation. The changes in backscattered light through the blood suspensions are then recorded versus time. The final aggregation time, corresponding to the reciprocal of the slope of the plot and calculated between 40 sec and 60 sec is expressed in seconds and corresponds to the evaluations of the rates of "rouleaux " formation. In addition, the apparatus enables one to investigate the shear rate required for the disaggregation of red cell suspensions. This can be performed as follows : the blood sample is sequentially submitted to decreasing shear rates ranging from 600 s–1 to 7 s–1 ; each shear rate being followed by a lag-time of 5 sec. This leads to the plot of the reflected flux versus shear rate, illustrating a critical shear rate below which the reflected flux tends to decrease. This phenomenon indicates that the shear rate applied to the aggregates is not enough to allow the dispersion of red blood cell aggregates. From this shear rate, one can define [22, 23] the critical shear stress necessary to induce the dispersion of the red cell aggregates. The disaggregation shear rate is expressed in sec–1.

Another apparatus (Myrenne aggregameter AMM1) [24] has been also used in order to investigate the kinetic of erythrocyte aggregation. This technique allows the analysis of the optical changes of the blood (its increase in light transmission) in a transparent cone-plate-chamber. The measuring principle can be described as follows : the blood sample is first sheared at 600 s–1 and is then suddenly stopped or brought to a low shear rate of 3 s–1. The aggregate formation in both cases in accompanied by an increase in light transmission. From the plot of the transmitted light as a function of time, the area below the curve in the first 10 seconds subsequent to flow stop or reducing flow is calculated and is respectively called M1 and M2. These parameters are related to the extent of red cell aggregation and have been shown [24] to be fairly well correlated with the rate constant of the aggregation process. The value of M2 is higher than M1 because of the increased probability of the red cell interaction at a low shear rate which leads to a more accelerated aggregation rate than that of red cell aggregation at rest.

All the measurements have been made at the ambiant temperature of the laboratory (22+–2°C) in the hour after blood sampling with the exception of plasma viscosity (37°C) and of red cell aggregation by Sefam erythroaggregameter (37°C).

The blood samples were collected before and after 30 days of treatment by *Ruscus* extract or placebo, from the veins of the legs before and after 10 minutes of venous stasis with a hyperpressure of 10 mmHg controlled by plethysmography.

Statistical analysis

Differences in mean values between different parameters and different groups were assessed by the Student's t-test.

Results

Hematocrit (Table I)

Before treatment, the controls did not have a significant increase in the hematocrit value, regardless of the hemodynamic conditions (at rest and after stasis). By contrast, the patients had a significant increase of the hematocrit values after stasis. After treatment, we observed that the placebo group always had a significant increase of the hematocrit value, but the *Ruscus* extract group did not exhibit an increase of the hematocrit after stasis.

Fibrinogen (Table I)

Before treatment, the fibrinogen concentration of the two groups of patients is significantly higher than that of the control subjects. The venous stasis did not significantly increase the fibrinogen level in the veins of the legs of the control subjects (2.71+–0.23), but in the patient groups, the venous stasis was accompanied with an increase of fibrinogen level although the increase was not significant. After treatment for the two groups of patients, no modification in the fibrinogen concentration was observed, before and after stasis.

Plasma viscosity (Table I)

Before treatment and at rest, the plasma viscosity was increased significantly for the two groups of patients in comparison with the control subjects. After stasis, the plasma viscosity was not modified in the control group, but significantly increased in the patient groups. After treatment, before and after stasis, the placebo group showed no modification of the plasma viscosity values. The group of patients treated with *Ruscus* extract had a significant improvement of plasma viscosity after stasis in comparison to their plasma viscosity before treatment in the same hemodynamic conditions and in comparison to the placebo group (1.45+–0.02 versus 1.32+–0.02 p<0.01; 1.41+–0.02 versus 1.32+–0.02 p<0.01). Thus patients receiving *Ruscus* extract had plasma viscosity before and after stasis comparable to that to the controls, i.e. the stasis is not accompanied by an increase in plasma viscosity.

Table I. – Evolution of hematocrit, fibrinogen, plasma viscosity before and after venous stasis in control subjects and in two groups of patients suffering from venous insufficiency before and after treatment with *Ruscus* extract or placebo. Measurements on blood samples collected in veins of legs at rest and after controlled venous stasis. Results are expressed as mean + – SEM. *p<0.05, **p<0.01, ***p<0.001.

	Before Treatment		After Treatment	
	At rest	After stasis	At rest	After stasis
Hematocrit %				
Controls n=20	42.5±0.8	43.4±0.9		
Placebo n=12	40.4±0.9 —*— 43.8±0.8		41.4±0.7 —*— 44.5±1	
Ruscus extract n=13	41±0.7 —*— 43.9±1.4		41.2±0.8	42.4±1
Fibrinogen g/l				
Controls n=20	2.41±0.17	2.71±0.23		
Placebo n=12	*— 2.81±0.3	*— 3.31±0.4	2.81±0.2	3.1±0.17
Ruscus extract n=13	3.30±0.1	3.54±0.15	3.14±0.14	3.26±0.11
Plasma viscosity mPa.s				
Controls n=20	1.29±0.02	1.31±0.018		
Placebo n=12	*— 1.34±0.02	*** — 1.42±0.03	1.35±0.02 —**— 1.41±0.02	
Ruscus extract n=13	1.33±0.02	**— 1.45±0.02	1.30±0.01 —**— 1.32±0.02	

Red cell deformability (Table II)

Before treatment and at rest, the red cell deformability index was identical in the control group and in the patients groups. After venous stasis, the red cell deformability index in the two patient groups was significantly higher than in control subjects. After treatment, the patients receiving placebo did not exhibit an appreciable modification and after stasis, the red blood deformability index was always significantly increased. The patients treated with *Ruscus* extract, before and after stasis, showed a normalization of this red cell parameter. The red cell deformability index in the patient group of *Ruscus* extract treatment was comparable to that of the control subjects.

Red cell aggregation-disaggregation (Table II)

High shear rate (600 s–1)

Before treatment, the red blood cell aggregation index, before stasis, was significantly higher in the two groups of patients than in the control group. Whereas the venous stasis did not modify this aggregation index in the control group, in the two patient groups, the venous stasis was accompanied by a significant increase in the aggregation index. After treatment, for the placebo group, the RBC aggregation index was not modified before and after venous stasis. By contrast, patients treated with *Ruscus* extract present a significant improvement of this index, especially after venous stasis, the patient group has a red blood cell aggregation index similar to that of the control subjects.

Low shear rate (3 s–1).

Before treatment for the two patient groups, the red blood cell aggregation indices were significantly increased in comparison to those of the control subjects. The venous stasis was also accompanied by an increase, which was not always significant. After treatment, patients receiving *Ruscus* extract had a significant improvement and decrease in the red blood cell aggregation regardless of the hemodynamic conditions (at rest, after stasis); whereas in the placebo group the values were unchanged. At low shear rate, the red blood cell aggregation index, at rest and after stasis, was similar to control in the patients treated with *Ruscus* extract.

Aggregation time (Table II)

Before treatment, at rest, patients with varicose veins had a significant decrease of the aggregation time in comparison with the control subjects. The venous stasis was accompanied by a significant acceleration of the red blood cell aggregation, whereas this was not seen in the control group. After treatment the red blood cell aggregation was not modified at rest and after venous stasis in the controls; by contrast, in the treated group, before and after stasis, the red blood cell aggregation time was improved significantly (21.75+–4.6 versus 27.8+–3.7 at rest) (17.2+–4.3 versus 25.7+–4.1 after stasis). The venous stasis unlike in the placebo group, was not accompanied by an acceleration of the red blood cell aggregation

Table II. – Evolution of red cell deformability index, kinetic indices of red cell aggregation, red cell aggregation time and red cell disaggregation shear rate before and after venous stasis in control subjects and in two groups of patients suffering from venous insufficiency before and after treatment with or placebo. Measurements on blood samples collected in veins of legs at rest and after controlled venous stasis. Results are expressed as mean ±SEM, *p<0.5, **p<0.02, ***p<0.01, ****p<0.001.

	Before treatment		After treatment	
	At rest	After stasis	At rest	After stasis
Red cell deformability				
Controls n=20	10.05±0.5	—10.8±0.6 **		
Placebo n=12	10.6±0.5 —**— 12.4±0.4		10.1±0.6—**—12.2±0.7 ***	
Ruscus extract n=13	10.9±0.5 —**— 12.8±0.6		9.56±0.4 ***	9.7±0.4
Red cell aggregation (after shear rate 600 s–1)				
Controls n=20	*** 6.08±0.65	6.28±0.62 ****		
Placebo n=12	8.92±0.67- ***— 11.2±0.7		9.07±0.58- ***—12.3±0.6 ****	
Ruscus extract n=13	8.51±0.77- ***—10.8±0.63		6.67±0.52 ****	7.12±0.62
Red cell aggregation (at low shear rate 3 s–1)				
Controls n=20	*** 8.44±0.7	9.4±0.82 ***		
Placebo n=12	11.45±0.9	12.63±1.1	10.8±0.7 —**— 12.1±0.9 *	*
Ruscus extract n=13	11..88±1.1— *—13.47±1.04		9.49±0.6 ***	10.53±0.8
Red cell aggregation time (sec)				
Controls n=20	*** 32.5±7	30.2±4 ***		
Placebo n=12	25.5±4 —**—19.4±3.8		23.9±4.6 — * — 20.2±4.5	
Ruscus extract n=13 25.7±4.1	21.75±4.6—**— 17.2±4.3		27.8±3.7 ***	25.7±4.1
Red cell disaggregation shear rate (sec–1)				
Controls n=20	*** 51.34±5.5	62.6±7 ***		
Placebo n=12	74.4±6 —**—82.9±5		72.4±4.9	79.9±6
Ruscus extract n=13	74.04±5.2—**—83.4±5.5		65.8±5.2 **	70.3±5.3

Red cell disaggregation shear rate (Table II)

Before treatment, the patients had a significant increase of red blood cell disaggregation shear rate, at rest; the aggregates of red cell were barely dissociable. After venous stasis, these aggregates were less dissociable, and venous stasis was accompanied by a deleterious effect on the red blood cell aggregates. In control subjects, venous stasis was not accompanied by an increase of red blood cell disaggregation threshold. After treatment, in the placebo group, the red blood cell aggregates were barely dissociable, but in the *Ruscus* extract group, the red blood cell disaggregation shear rate was not disturbed by venous stasis and significantly improved (although not normalized).

Discussion

The viscosity of whole blood depends on the flow velocity or on the shear rates and on the shear stresses. In the post-capillary venules as well as in small veins, the first contribution to blood viscosity in the red cell aggregation-disaggregation phenomenon. The second factor controlling blood viscosity is the cellular concentration or hematocrit. The third factor is the plasma viscosity which depends on the plasma proteins (e.g. fibrinogen, albumin).

The lowest shear rates are found at the venous side of the circulation; this shear rate coincides with the red cell aggregation [8, 3, 25, 26]. If there is a dilatation of vessels (varicose veins), this shear rate can be decreased and become very low if not completely null. In the same time, proteins as albumin can pass through the venule or vein wall and lead to an hemoconcentration resulting in an increase of fibrinogen level and an increase of red blood cells. It is this foreseeable that the red cell-red cell or red cell-endothelial cell interactions will be influenced depending on the modifications of red blood cell properties and of the plasma proteins.

In the present study, the results show that patients with varicose veins of the legs have significant disturbances of the main hemorheological parameters of the blood viscosity, and that stasis on the varicose vein side aggravates these microrheological disturbances and thus blood viscosity.

Ruscus extract treatment is accompanied by an improvement of several microrheological factors of blood viscosity; in fact it seems that *Ruscus* extract treatment leads to :

— a significant decrease in hemoconcentration mainly under conditions of venous stasis (hematocrit, plasma viscosity); this could be explained by effects on resistance vessels and the permeability of capillaries, venules and veins, or by an effect on interstitiel conjunctive and vascular tissue by anti-edema effect.

— an improvement of red cell deformability, and inhibition of the delete-rious effect of venous stasis.

— an improvement of the tendency of the red blood cells to hyperaggregate, especially at low shear rates and even after venous stasis.

Thus, the clinical activity of *Ruscus* extract probably is due to facilitating the return of blood, decreasing the hemoconcentration in stasis, and opposing the hyperaggregation tendency of red cells and the adhesiveness of these cells to the vessel wall.

Our result confirm previous studies done *in vitro* as well as earlier clinical studies [27, 28]. A therapeutic improvement of the microcirculation and of the hemorheological properties of blood appear to be of importance in the disturbances of venous circulation.

References

1. Lowe GDO. Blood rheology and venous thrombosis. Clinical Hemorheology. 1984; 4: 571-588.
2. Chien S., Usami S, Dellenback RJ, *et al.* Blood viscosity : influence of erythrocyte aggre-gation. Science 1967; 157 : 829-831.
3. Chien S, Sung LA. Bases physicochimiques et implications cliniques de l'agrégation des globules rouges. Hémorhéologie et agrégation érythrocytaire. Ed. EM Inter Paris, 1986; 122-147.
4. Schmid Schonbein H, Gallasch G, Volger E, Microrheology and protein chemistry of pa-thological red cell aggregation (blood sludge) studied *in vitro*. Biorheology 1973 ; 10 : 213-227.
5. Meril EW, Gilliland ER, Lee TS, *et al.* Blood rheology : effects of fibrinogen deduced by addition. Circ Res 1966; 18 : 437-446.
6. Wells RE, Garowski TH, Cox PJ, *et al.* Influence of fibrinogen on flow properties of ery-throcyte suspensions. Am J Physiol 1964; 207 : 1035-1040.
7. Brooks DE, Greig R, Jansen J. Mechanisms of erythrocyte aggregation Erythrocyte me-chanics and blood flow. *In* : Cokelet GR, Meiselman HK, Brooks DE (Ed), New York, AR Lise Inc., 1980; 119-140.
8. Chien S. Biophysical behaviour of red cells in suspensions. The red blood cell, 2nd edi-tion, edited by D. Mac N. Surgenor, Academic Press, New York, 1975, 2 : 1031.
9. Goldsmith HL. Blood flow and thrombosis. Throm Hemost. 1974; 32 : 35-48.
10. Goldsmith HL, Karino T. Mechanically induced thromboemboli. Quantitative cardiovas-cular studies, clinical and research applications of engineering principles. Edited by Hwang NHC, Gross DR, Patel DJ, Baltimore, University Park Press, 1979; 289-351.

11. Chien S. Blood rheology and its relation to flow resistance and transcapillary exchanges with special reference to shock. Adv Microcir 1969; 2 : 89.

12. Schmid Schonbein H. Critical closing pressure of yield shear stress as the cause of disturbed peripheral circulation. Acta Chir Scand 1976; 10 : sup. 465, 142.

13. Lerche D, Klaus H, Kunter H. Study of aggregation of human red blood cells. Stud Bioph 1976; 56 : 21.

14. Volger E, Schmid Shonbein H, Gosen J, *et al.* Microrheology and light transmission of blood. IV. The kinetics of artificial red cell aggregation induced by Dextran. Pflügers Arch 1975; 354 : 319.

15. Farhaeus R. The suspension stability of blood. Physiol Rev 1929; 9 : 241.

16. Chien S, Usami S, Dellenback RJ, *et al.* Shear dependent interaction of plasma proteins with erythrocytes in blood rheology. Am J Physiol. 1970; 219 : 143.

17. International Committee for Standardization in Haematology. Guidelines for measurement of blood viscosity and erythrocyte deformability. Clinical Hemorheology 1986; 6 : 439-453.

18. Caen J, Larrieu MJ, Samama M. L'hémostase : méthode d'exploration et diagnostic pratique. L'expension scientifique, Paris 1975.

19. Jung F, Roggenkamp HG, Schreider R, *et al.* Ein neues gerät zur quantifizierung der blutplasma-viskosität. Biomed Tech 1983; 28 : 249-252.

20. Hanss M. Erythrocyte filterability measurement by the initial flow rate method. Biorheology 1983; 20 : 199-211.

21. Donner M, Siadat M, Stoltz JF. Erythrocyte aggregation : approach by light scattering determination. Biorheology 1988; 25 : 367-375.

22. Othmane A, Bitbol M, Snabre P, *et al.* Red cell aggregation in insulin-dependent diabetics. Clinical Hemorheology 1989; 9 : 281-295.

23. Snabre P, Bitbol M, Mills P. Cell disaggregation behaviour in shear flow. Biophys J 1987; 51 : 795-807.

24. Schmid Schonbein H, Volger E, Teitel P, *et al.* New hemorheological technics for the routine laboratory. Clinical hemorheology 1982; 2 : 93-105.

25. Stoltz JF. L'agrégation érythrocytaire : aspects thérapeutiques. Hémorhéologie et agrégation érythrocytaire. Ed EM Inter Paris, 1986; 164-171.

26. Quemada D. Rheology of concentrated disperse system. A model for non newtonian shear viscosity in steady flows. Rheol Acta 1978; 17 : 632-642.

27. Kiesewetter H, Blume J, Scheffler P, *et al.* Efficacité clinique de Cyclo 3 Fort associé à la contention dans les insuffisances veineuses chroniques des membres inférieurs. Gazette Médicale 1987; tome 94 : 10, 2-7.

28. Kiesewetter H. *In vitro* testung der rheologischen Wirkkomponente des *Ruscus*-Präparates Phlebodril. Interner Bericht, 1984.

Authors index

IMPRIMERIE LOUIS-JEAN
BP 87 — 05003 GAP Cedex
Tél. : 92.51.35.23
Dépôt légal : 230 — Mars 1991
Imprimé en France